## Description of
## Elisabeth Haich's painting on the cover

If we cultivate spiritual awareness and attain the universal consciousness, we acquire mastery over the 7 natural forces which,
when harnessed to pull in one direction, can carry us to the goal
with incredible swiftness.
The picture symbolizes this state. The figure representing the
spirit is standing in the triumphal chariot. One hand is radiating the
power which directs the natural forces. In the left hand is held a
prayer wheel such as is used in Tibet and which symbolizes unity
with the Divine. The horses race with this figure to the goal where
we achieve the perfection which Christ intimated to us in the words:
"Be ye therefore perfect, even as your Father which is in Heaven
is perfect."

*Elisabeth Haich 1976*

D0881817

# Sexual Energy and Yoga

By Elisabeth Haich
INIATION
WISDOM OF THE TAROT
THE DAY WITH YOGA

By Elisabeth Haich and Selvarajan Yesudian
RAJA YOGA
YOGA AND DESTINY
YOGA AND HEALTH

# SEXUAL ENERGY AND YOGA

## by Elisabeth Haich

translated by D. Q. Stephenson

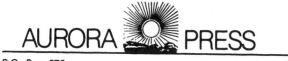

AURORA PRESS

P.O. Box 573

Santa Fe, N.M. 87504

© Elisabeth Haich 1982

No part of this book may be reproduced by any mechanical, photographic or electronic process, or in the form of a phonographic recording, nor may it be stored in a retrieval system, transmitted, translated into another language, or otherwise copied for public or private use, excepting brief passages quoted for purposes of review, without the permission of the publisher.

First published in 1982 by:
Aurora Press, Inc.
P.O. Box 573
Santa Fe, N.M. 87504
Printed in the United States of America
ISBN: 0-943358-03-5
Library of Congress Catalogue No: 74-83158

I dedicate this book to
those ambitious people who demand the best
of life and of themselves

ELISABETH HAICH
AND
SELVARAJAN
YESUDIAN
With Mrs. Haich's
painting and sculpture
Zurich, Switzerland
1981
© Barbara Somerfield

# Contents

# FACTS ABOUT ELISABETH HAICH

Elisabeth Haich, March 20, 1897-July 31, 1994, was the second of four children born into an upper middle class family in Budapest, Hungary. Even as a young child, her unique gifts were expressed as a pianist, painter and sculptress. Her sculptures are exhibited in Hungary, as monuments and in plazas. She was married and had one son who later joined her in teaching Yoga in Switzerland. In close connection with Selvarajan Yesudian, she began giving Yoga lectures in 1939.

At the end of World War II, she was forced to leave Hungary with the assistance of Selvarajan Yesudian and resettled in Switzerland where she lived until the end of her life. In cooperation with Yesudian, she began the oldest and largest Yoga school in Europe.

In 1953 Elisabeth Haich wrote her bestselling book, *Initiation*, which has been translated into seventeen languages with millions of copies sold worldwide. Her other books include, *The Day With Yoga, Sexual Energy and Yoga, Wisdom of the Tarot* and authored with Selvarajan Yesudian, *Self Healing Yoga and Destiny*. All of these titles are published by Aurora Press in English.

Until the end of her life, Elisabeth Haich lectured and counseled seekers.

# Illustrations

# Preface

In theoretical research and psychotherapeutic practice modern depth psychologists have inevitably been brought into contact with mythology and religion and have come to see and understand legends and fairy tales in terms of their discipline. They have likewise extended their research to include the mysticism and alchemy of the Middle Ages and have also found many points of contact with eastern philosophies and religions. The relationship between Yoga and depth psychology is particularly clear.

All the same, the many and various identities between depth psychology and Yoga have led depth psychologists to different conclusions. Some place depth psychology and Yoga more or less on a par, others try to understand experience acquired through Yoga and meditation in terms of the symbolism of depth psychology, and others again even attempt to explain Yoga by means of depth psychology.

J. H. Schultz finds many points in common between the highest level of autogenous training and Raja Yoga. He also believes that a comparison of their own technique with that of Hatha Yoga is particularly instructive for practitioners of autogenous training. The passive exercises in the lying and sitting posture of autogenous training are paralleled by two asanas of Hatha Yoga, the basic sitting posture and the dead posture. On the other hand Schultz believes there is no connection between autogenous training and the Hatha Yoga exercises involving movement and Yoga breathing. Schultz hopes through autogenous training to annex the actual substance of Yoga exactly in the same way as, he believes, the actual substance of mystic magnetism has been annexed by rational hypnotherapy.

Autogenous training, however, is not really a method which has

13

scientifically pinpointed and evaluated the true nature of Hatha or Raja Yoga but is rather a Yoga which is incompletely understood. Autogenous training will be able to annex the actual substance of Hatha Yoga and Raja Yoga only if it itself becomes Yoga. It must be remembered in this connection that, although there are various paths of Yoga, that is to say, various forms of Yoga, Yoga has but one aim.

Even as a half-understood form of Yoga autogenous training is one of the greatest blessings of modern psychotherapy. What a blessing, then, a fully understood Yoga would be for depth psychology and psychotherapy!

Langen holds that the highest states of consciousness attained through Yoga exercises and meditation are forms of hypnosis. We believe it is perfectly right for Yoga and meditation to be included with due care in the scope of research in depth psychology. But it would be wrong for investigators to attempt to explain the phenomena of Yoga and meditation in terms of depth psychology in its present state. This would lead to false conclusions. Instead the investigators must first meditate and perform Yoga exercises themselves for some years and then try to describe what they have experienced.

After such research the depth psychologists would be in a position to distinguish between states of expanded consciousness and states of reduced consciousness. They would also have a clearer understanding of the phenomena which they all at present ascribe to hypnosis.

At the beginning of the age of depth psychology the existence of the unconscious mind was denied by many psychiatrists in the light of their theoretical knowledge. Anyone who at that time had witnessed the power of the unconscious in himself and in patients could only greet this denial with a smile. It is rather the same today when we read psychological treatises on Yoga and meditation. To practise Yoga and meditation for some time is to realize clearly the difference between the present state of depth psychology and Yoga. For the highest stages of Yoga exercises and meditation are not hypnotic states with a reduced or restricted consciousness but states of the very highest consciousness with a vast expansion of awareness.

Jung called depth analysis in psychology the modern form of

initiation. The inner spiritual processes taking place during analysis are compared by him to the development a man experiences before and during initiation. Jung considers that the great eastern philosophers are symbolic psychologists. The 'diamond body' of the East and the 'resurrected body' of Christians strike him as curious psychological facts. He also regards the whole of medieval alchemy as psychological symbolism. Jung speaks of the self and the way to the self; he speaks of Christ as the archetype.

Jung is certainly right when he holds that what is called metaphysical must be accessible to mental experience otherwise it could have no effect at all on mankind. Jung formulates no propositions concerning the metaphysical but describes forms in which the metaphysical can be experienced. For him these forms are the symbols.

It therefore remains an open question whether the self of which he speaks is the same as the self of Yoga. It remains an open question whether the 'archetype Christ' is the same as the 'living Christ'.

Jung compares religious and philosophical ideas from the East and West from the standpoint of psychological symbolism and finds there are marked differences. For example, he compares the 'sorrow-laden hero Christ' with the 'golden flower' of the East or contrasts the 'historical personal Christ' with the saying of the Eastern sage Hui Ming King: 'Without coming into being, without passing away, without past, without future.'

These comparisons, however, are not just, for Jung has compared forms of expression from different levels of knowledge. If comparisons are to be made, the comparisons in East and West must be made at the same level of knowledge. In a proper comparison the equivalent of the 'golden flower' of the East is the 'rosy cross' in the West. The counterpart of the words of Hui Ming King is then Christ's saying: 'Before Abraham was, I am.'

We believe that if legitimate comparisons are made, no difference will be found between what the East and the West want to say.

The essential difference between Jung's understanding of the matter and our own is that we believe that the bounds of the metaphysical accessible to mental experience are very much wider for the man who practises Yoga and meditates than for the man whose approach to the metaphysical is through the concepts of depth psychology.

Yoga and meditation or the exercises of the Rosicrucians open up to mental experience metaphysical realms which are closed to the depth psychologist.

The descriptions given by oriental sages of their experience in Yoga and meditation are not symbols for psychological experience but are the very experience itself. Neither the 'diamond body' of the East nor the 'resurrected body' of the Christian West is a symbol for a psychological fact but is this fact itself. And alchemy is not limited merely to describing the happenings of depth psychology but describes a process of development taking place in man's body and soul which leads in actual fact and not symbolically to the coming to consciousness of the spirit in the resurrected body.

Depth psychologists owe Jung an enormous debt for having shown them the way to oriental wisdom, to Yoga, and to meditation. It simply remains for the depth psychologists to tread this path themselves.

To avoid misunderstanding let us stress that we do not wish to oppose Yoga to modern depth psychology. It is simply a matter of maintaining the correct relationship between the two. In reality Yoga is superordinate to depth psychology. It is not Yoga that is contained in depth psychology but depth psychology that is contained in Yoga. Yoga must point the way for the future research of depth psychologists. For Yoga contains everything that can be said about the unconscious, the conscious and the supraconscious. But in investigating these propositions the investigators must not proceed from theoretical assumptions but acquire experience by performing the exercises themselves.

It is impossible to perform Yoga exercises regularly and for any length of time without a confrontation with oneself in the sense of modern depth psychology. Devotees of Yoga who imagine they can proceed along the path of Yoga without having to confront their own unconscious mind are greatly mistaken. Yoga exercises are good for men and women; through them they become healthier, more vital and capable of greater achievement. But for everyone who does Yoga and meditates there comes a point in his inner development where the confrontation with his own personal unconscious becomes inescapable. If this confrontation fails to

PREFACE

materialize, then even the Yoga practitioner is afflicted by a neurosis.

On the other hand everyone who practises the methods of depth psychology will one day undergo experiences which transcend the bounds of the depth psychology we know and are only describable in Yoga.

Yoga and depth psychology both aim to expand the conscious mind. In the depth psychologist's treatment of a neurosis unconscious material which according to the normal circumstances of life properly belongs to the conscious mind is raised to the conscious level. That is to say, in healing neuroses by psychotherapy the conscious mind is restored to its normal condition.

The performance of Yoga exercises also makes unconscious material conscious. But with Yoga exercises and meditation the human consciousness can be extended beyond the normal bounds to a higher state of consciousness.

Anyone who has learnt in psychological work how to make unconscious material conscious will already know something about the method of raising the conscious mind to a higher level of consciousness. The patient who has been cured of a neurosis by psychotherapy is thus better able to develop his consciousness than an average person for whom the idea of growing awareness is somewhat foreign. The experience he has had to go through in overcoming the neurosis may make a man understand the process of the gradual development of human consciousness and induce him to promote this development by a conscious effort.

Here no doubt we find the deeper significance for mankind of the psychological knot we call a neurosis. And here too is the deeper significance of the work of the psychotherapist who helps in the development of consciousness.

In this book Elisabeth Haich shows what sexual energy really is and how through Yoga this energy can be converted into the highest consciousness. Sexuality and the highest consciousness are two different forms in which the one divine creative force, the Logos, is manifested. Sexual energy, the lowest form of the Logos, can in man become the highest form of the Logos, divine consciousness.

In the description of this transformation of energies it is quite clear that Yoga also embraces the spiritual processes which we today refer to as depth psychology. But at the same time it is quite obvious how far Yoga transcends modern depth psychology.

Elisabeth Haich warns against trying to skip stages of consciousness. She shows how the power of sexual energy can be recognized and how sexuality must first be experienced before it can be transformed. The author also describes the abnormal reactions and disturbances that may ensue if anyone attempts to put his consciousness through a process of development for which he is not yet mature. Here we are confronted with the whole modern psychology of the unconscious.

The author then goes on to describe stages in the development of consciousness which are still unknown to depth psychologists. Even the magical powers acquired through expanded consciousness are discussed and the nature of these powers is shown.

Reading this book makes us aware that Freud intuitively grasped the true nature of sexuality. Throughout his life he struggled with the concept of the libido and continually reformulated it. In his view it was to be understood not only in the narrow sense of sexuality but also in a much wider and more comprehensive sense.

Freud also saw that sexuality can be transformed into spiritually creative power and called this process sublimation.

However, sublimation and the process which Elisabeth Haich calls transformation of sexual energy are not the same. Freud saw sublimation as the possibility of being able to deal meaningfully with sexuality without repression. The sexual energy transformed by Yoga on the other hand will lead man to the highest form of consciousness.

Even so it was Freud's genius that saw in the 'libido' and 'sublimation' the energies and potentialities which are vital and necessary for the development of human consciousness.

Growing consciousness is the purpose of human life, and the highest consciousness is the goal of human development. This development proceeds stepwise from man the creature of unconscious impulses to the fully conscious God-man.

Modern depth psychology can help us along a part of this path of development but only Yoga and meditation can bring us to the goal.

H. S.

# Introduction

In writing this book I have felt free to express my thoughts in simple terms and have therefore retained the old, not yet hackneyed words, without using new, scientific-sounding ones for concepts already named in the oldest books of mankind. Thus the primal source of all life, which no scientist can explain, is designated by the old word 'God'. If we think of new words in order to prevent people from clinging to their old erroneous interpretations of that word, then they will transfer their misconceptions to the meaning of the new words. To fight against ignorance is futile. Those, however, who sense a true concept of God behind the so-called modern terms, will also perceive it in the old word 'God'. Why should we therefore change the words? We may be satisfied if, in the very depths of our soul, we can have a humble, reverent intimation of God. Through rational knowledge we cannot reach God. Knowledge, recognition can be attained only by comparison – through the tree of knowledge of good and evil – but God cannot be compared to anything, to anything at all. Therefore we can never recognize God, we can never know what God is, we can only *be* God.

Men of science take painstaking care to avoid the use of this concept and word 'God'. We sense their fear that in the final analysis it might not sound scholarly enough if they were to use the simple word 'God'. This fear, however, is only common to those who are not real, genuine scholars. For if Spinoza, Newton or Einstein, for instance, through the science of mathematics, came to find and accept God as the primal cause of *all being*, and to accept his existence as proven, then it is with a good conscience that the ancient Biblical word 'God' can be retained in this book for the ultimate origin of origins. This word, then, is used here not in a religious-sentimental sense, but in line with the usage of Spinoza, Newton and Einstein. We are content if the reader experiences the same deep devotion, reverence and humility before this word as was felt by these greatest scholars of all time. In these feelings the simple man meets with the truly great man of science, just as in the Biblical account the simple shepherds met with the magicians at the highest level of knowledge. We have therefore attempted to express matters in such a way that they will be understood equally well by the simple 'shepherds' and by the 'magician'.

The word 'love' also presented me with a problem. Since there are various expressions in the Hungarian language for the various manifestations of love, we Hungarians cannot understand how the same word 'love' can be used to describe one's feelings for God, one's parents, a child, one's native country, sweetheart, neighbour, but also for a dog or a horse. In Hungarian there are different expressions for all these different kinds of love, and these clearly show *why* and *whom* we love. For the understanding of this book, however, it is very important that we correctly understand the various feelings of love. Thus, in order to avoid misunderstanding I had to clarify these different kinds of love by paraphrase. As a result, the text became more cumbersome than I could have wished. But I had no alternative.

Elsewhere too in this book, things will be mentioned for which there are no appropriate words in a Western language. Let us remember the difficulties that are involved in the mere accurate description of a dream. In the depths of the Self there are no dimensions, just as there is no concept of time, and frequently also no personal feeling. How can one then describe the experiences which take place in the depths of the soul and which we experience as pure states of being within us, if no appropriate words exist?

Therefore, it was exceedingly difficult for me to speak of concepts for which there is no good and apt translation in English or German, and yet more difficult to explain concepts for which here in the West there are no words at all. That is why it is impossible to translate, for instance, Sanskrit, Chinese, Tibetan or Hungarian texts into Western languages. One is therefore left with the necessity of paraphrase. But in spite of all efforts to make states of being comprehensible through words, these descriptions remain only external representations of what happens. *They do not become states of being as long as the reader himself is not able to experience these descriptions within himself, in his spirit, as a state of being.* What is said here is equally valid for both sexes. Nevertheless, I have generally only referred to the male, since it would have been too laborious to repeat the same thing each time for the female. In order not to make the text unbearably cumbersome, I have chosen the 'crown of creation', man, to discuss the problems of sexuality. So that misunderstanding does not arise, however, I should like to emphasize that everything said in this book about sexuality and the development of consciousness, *applies as much to the female as to the male.*

This book, like every book on Yoga, only has genuine value if we put into practice what has been written and *try it out on ourselves.* No matter how beautifully we may describe the best and most nourishing foods and the most refreshing drinks to a hungry and thirsty man, and no matter how avidly he may read, and only read, these descriptions, he will never be sated. After reading the most beautiful books he will continue to be hungry and thirsty and to seek food and drink. Therefore we must practise Yoga and not only read about it! This is particularly true of this book, since it tries to reveal the deepest secrets of the higher level of Yoga. This secret of the higher level of Yoga is the stimulation and use of the latent nerve and brain centres, which are the seat of the spiritual centres, termed *chakras* in the philosophy of Yoga, and the use of the only fuel absolutely indispensable for this purpose – sexual energy. But we leave it to the person who seeks and desires to find the ultimate sources of life to put that secret into practice, to test the truth of it on ourselves, to learn and derive immense profit from it. The hungry and thirsty must themselves eat and drink!

My final and perhaps most important point is that this book can only be a real guide to those people who, moved by an unquenchable thirst for God, wish to tread the steep path to the kingdom of heaven. Those who take this path because they lack the courage for the outer and inner struggles of life cannot profit from my instructions. For those people, too, who for some reason cannot attain a life in the world – which is what they really desire above all else – therefore for those who have not yet passed through life in this world, and seek God only out of fear or helplessness, this book can at best offer curious reading matter or perhaps even an experiment.

Only for those who genuinely seek God does it have supreme significance, for as long as we cannot be children we cannot become adults. The childhood that we have not experienced draws us back!

My mother-tongue is an Asiatic primitive language and for this reason, as said already, many words have had to be paraphrased. My dear friends helped me to overcome these difficulties with endless patience and here also I wish to convey to them my most sincere gratitude. I wish to extend this gratitude in particular to Dr Helmut Speer, who enriched the book with a preface, and moreover gave me a number of valuable suggestions.

# Chapter 1

# What is Sexuality?

In God the two poles rest within each other in perfect unity and absolute equilibrium. In this state there is no tension but neither is there creation. Creation begins with the negative pole being expelled from this unity and the two poles consequently drawing apart and becoming opposed to each other as force and resistance. Yet be they never so far removed from each other, the unity between the two poles never ceases to exist; they belong to each other through all eternity: they can never be completely sundered, unity continues to subsist between them as a magical tension of infinite power which draws the two poles back to each other without intermission in order to restore the original condition of rest between them.

On this tension the whole of creation is borne. Without it no creation, no life, is possible, for this very tension *is* life. This means that every living creature contains these two poles within itself, as its vital self, otherwise it could not live at all. In man the seat of the positive pole is in the skull, and of the negative pole in the coccyx at the base of the spine, and the tension between the two constitutes life.

Life must be propagated in the new living creature, and for a new living creature to come into being, the two opposed poles must create between them a new vital tension out of which new life can be engendered. Even though every living creature, including man, bears this vital tension between the two poles in its spine, it nevertheless *manifests* in its body *only one pole*, which awaits conjunction with a contrary pole from outside before it can transmit life in a new living creature. In his physical consciousness as a human being, man has no inkling that he bears within his spirit, within his true self, these two poles. He identifies himself with his body, which under the present order of Nature, manifests only one pole and seeks completion from outside, from another person manifesting the opposite pole. The perfect unification of the two poles in the same body is impossible, for matter isolates, separates and offers resistance. Even so, the two poles strive for unity in and through the body and they seek a way of attaining rest in each other and at least of imitating the primal state. The two poles are manifested in the body in the two sexes by the genital organs which enable physical unity to be attained sexually for a short time. Since the repose of the two poles in each other is the primal state of God, of being, of life, the reunification of the two poles – the encounter of the two sexes – engenders a new tension, a new life, a new creature in a cell suited to the purpose. This in turn bears within itself the divine tension of life, but again manifests only one pole in its body – one sex – through which earthly life is transmitted by the recurrent union of the sexes. This is sexuality.

The energy which is manifested through sexuality and *which is the link between spirit and matter* and thus possesses the important faculty of *helping a spirit into the body*, of impregnating matter with new life, is called 'sexual energy'.

But, although man with his consciousness has fallen out of the paradisiacal primal state in which both poles repose in each other, he feels, although quite unconsciously, that such a primal state remains a possibility and, out of his knowledge of the manifested half, he yearns to be restored to the wholeness which he bears in his spirit, in his own life, which he himself always was, is, and will be. He does not realize that he can attain this primal state of conscious wholeness of his own being in his physical, earthly life, and still less does he realize that the only means capable of helping him to do this is his own sexual energy. Sexual energy, then, holds for man a secret which has nothing to do with the procreation of new life. *Just as sexual energy has helped man out of his spiritual state into the body, so it can help him to return in full awareness to his divine primal state of wholeness.*

At the same time this secret means that the attributes of sexual energy – if he does not expend this life-giving and life-creating power but retains it for his own body – can, on the one hand, replenish his body with life, enhance his inner vitality, keep him in the bloom of youth or regenerate him, and, on the other hand, by enhancing his vitality, wake, stimulate and activate his higher nerve and brain centres and arouse them out of their previously latent condition. These nerve plexuses and brain centres in the body serve to manifest and sustain the purely intellectual focuses which man bears in his spiritual being and which are termed *chakras* in the philosophy of Yoga. And if through the action of life-giving sexual energy which has not been expended but retained for his own body, these focuses or *chakras* are enabled to manifest themselves, then man attains mastery over the forces of Nature in his own being and, through his consciously developed hypnotic power of suggestion, in every living creature. He attains divine all-consciousness, he becomes a whole, an illuminate, a man of magic, a white magician.

This book is intended as an approach to the secret of how a human being can attain this level of universal consciousness with the aid of controlled sexual energy and how he can obtain mastery over natural forces. But not for everyone! For there are two kinds of people on earth. The living who are already 'human beings'. And the dead who are simply 'men' and 'women'.

The living, like the dead, carry a body with them – they *live* in a body – and since the human body under the present order of Nature manifests only one half of the whole, only one pole, the living, like the dead, bear in their body only one half of the whole, one pole, one sex. And so, although the living also have a body and perhaps lead a healthy sex life based on love, they are nevertheless aware that sexuality and all the problems arising from sexuality originate only in the body, belong only to the body and not to their true being, their spirit, their *self*. The spirit – the true Ego, also called the Self – has no sex, and consequently a human being who has attained consciousness in his spirit, in his true being, a human who is awake and alive, no longer seeks the half in everything but the whole, the absolute; no longer the transient, the physical, but the eternal, the divine. His problems do not stem from the sexuality of the body but, if at all, from the contrast between the earthly-physical and the spiritual-divine. His goal is to become conscious in spirit and to obtain complete mastery over the body and over all the forces at his disposal in his true being. In their consciousness these people stand above sexuality, above sex, and are already 'human beings' even if at a physical level they perhaps still lead a sex life. It is their aim to reach what the highest card of the tarot pack illustrates so vividly: the great Self, the great Ego, which no longer manifests sex, because it has consciously united the two sexes in itself and is consequently a whole, and lets the homunculus, which is a physical being and still belongs to a sex, dance on his hand like a little marionette, as an agent of manifestation, because its role in the earthly-material world so wishes.

The 'dead', still unconscious in spirit and leading a purely physical existence, who do not yet live themselves (only their body is alive), are at first still separate sexual beings and think only in terms of sex. They are still the tiny marionettes, the homunculi, which dance round on the palm of the great Ego and play their role. They are still only one half of the whole; they are first and foremost 'men' and 'women'. For them there exists only sex and nothing else. Even the other great instinct, self-preservation, exists for them solely as a servant of sensuality and sex; they eat, drink and indulge in dainties only so as to be as healthy as they can and to squeeze the last ounce of sexuality out of their bodies. Earning one's bread and butter, making money, succeeding in a career, making contact with other people, everything they say, tell, write and do, has only one motivating force: the sex drive. It is their supreme ambition and pride to attain the acme of sexual potency and amorous success. Of course, since they have never attained consciousness of spirit, they are left, once over-use saps their bodies, with nothing but their own infinite emptiness and, as their bodies decay, they are plunged into ever profounder darkness and senility. At birth their spirit died to the body and their consciousness lives and dies with the life and death of the body. Christ calls them 'the dead who bury their dead' and Paul says of them that they are 'the natural man [who] receiveth not the things of the Spirit of God: for they are foolishness unto him'. This book was not written for these people, for they would never understand it and would regard it as foolishness.

But there are 'people' who have seen that those who grow weak and senile with age are not the only inhabitants of the earth but that there have been at all times people who, as they have grown old, and often very old, have not become senile but have, from day to day, grown richer in mind, wiser, more knowledgeable, powerful and potent, and who, like Goethe for instance, have even preserved the beauty of their bodies. There are people who have already seen that there are two kinds of human beings on earth, let us call them, as we choose, the living and the dead, the wakeful and the sleepers, the conscious and the unconscious, and who have become dimly aware of the background of this difference and would like to follow these examples. It was for them that this book was written. For those who understand or would like to understand why Paul said: 'Why fearest thou Death, thou fool; we shall not all sleep but we shall all be changed!' That is to say, we do not all lose our consciousness in death. For all those who seek the path from the bondage of the body to the freedom of the spirit, this book was written.

We want to pass on to others the crystallized and clarified results of the ancient philosophy of Yoga and the observations and experience we have garnered during several decades. This experience was not derived from books, not affected by the various ingeniously conceived scientific theses that change every ten years, but, free from all imposed influences, has been discovered, experienced and felt on our own path through life.

It is important at this stage to stress one point in particular. Just as no two people are the same, so no two paths are identical. Human destinies vary enormously, and so do the paths we all follow to the final goal. It is extremely rare for two people of opposite sexes to come together, for each to be the complement of the other in perfect harmony, and for both to achieve a truly gladdening oneness. But it is rarer still for two people who have captured this wonderful togetherness to maintain it throughout a lifetime till they are parted by death. And so if two people have been vouchsafed God's exceptional gift of a life spent together in such inner harmony, let them enjoy this rare union and be grateful. If this book should fall into their hands, they may rest assured it is not meant for them. Yet they should remember that there are many of their fellow human beings who perhaps also once found a similar sense of belongingness but, through force of circumstances, lost it again very soon afterwards and remained alone. And there are many, very many, who never at any time in their lives have found such a bond but must lead a life of loneliness from beginning to end, as if God wanted to show that the answer to their problem must be sought and found not in personal relations but in some other way. For these and others who feel a deep inner urge to seek and find God this book may be a help and a guide.

It is not our intention to wean aspirants to the path of Yoga away from a *healthy* human attitude towards earthly life and earthiy love. Indeed, the very opposite is true: what we want to do is to induce such an attitude in everyone, for our path must and can start only in health. But Yoga is the healthiest and therefore the shortest path of development by which human beings advance to the highest goal, to God.

This path, starting from the first awakening, from the deepest, dimmest, still semi-feral level of consciousness and progressing to perfect self-knowledge, to divine self-awareness, and true oneness with God, we call Yoga.

And since the driving force which helps man to tread this path, to climb ever farther and higher along it, and indeed even impels him, and manifests itself at its lowest level in the body, where it represents the link between mind and matter, is sexual energy, *Yoga and sexual energy cannot be separated from each other.*

To tread the path of Yoga does not mean that we must embrace an abstemious life. At the beginning of the Yoga path we must first learn how to live healthily in every way, *with* Nature and not *against* Nature. This includes healthy eating and drinking and, of course, a healthy erotic life. Yoga teaches us how one first becomes healthy in mind, in spirit, and thus in body, and how one lives healthily. How can one give up sex life if he has never yet known what a healthy sex life means?

The later stages at which one grows out of the body more and more into the spirit would be attained by everyone in any case as a natural development of the conscious mind, for this development is inherent in us just as a plant or flower contains the process whereby it first takes root, then puts out leaves, produces flowers, and finally reaches the climax when it brings forth fruit because this goal was always latent in the seed. And man, too, carries within him like seed the ability to reach the highest goal – God – and to become a God-man. Following the natural laws, however, this path of natural development takes a very long time, perhaps thousands of years; it is laborious and fraught with sorrows, and may need many reincarnations. But man bears a secret faculty within himself, in his own sexual energy, by which he can realize this development and evolution in a much shorter time. Just as one can use artificial means of forcing flowers so that they blossom much earlier than they would in Nature, so man can achieve maturity much earlier on his inward path to consciousness with the various methods of Yoga which quicken our inner development. None of the stages of development may be omitted but time can be shortened like a telescope. As the flower needs extra warmth for this process, so man also needs extra warmth and vitality kindled by the secret fire. And the fuel – the secret fire of the Rosicrucians – is, as we have said, sexual energy. Between the natural kind of development and the development quickened by sexual energy there is, however, a very great difference. It does not reside merely in the fact that the goal, universal consciousness, is attained much more quickly but also in the fact that man, during the time he is learning about this possibility and putting it into practice, is still in possession of his full sexual potency, and is capable not only of covering the path of spiritual development much more expeditiously but also, and at the same time, of laying hold of the vitalizing force latent in sexual energy, of converting it into divine creative power, and of subjugating it to his ends. Hence the name of this system: Yoga or 'yoke'. These powers also endow man concomitantly with magical abilities which have often been described and which are familiar to us from the lives of great saints and yogis – known in the terminology of Yoga as *siddhis* – such as clairvoyance, regeneration of one's own body, miraculous healing, the casting out of demons, the resurrection of the dead, levitation, telepathy and prophecy, and so forth.

In one single life this supreme goal is achieved only by those who bring with them from previous existences a nervous system with the stamina needed to endure the last and most difficult cycle of the path and the high frequencies of the ever-mounting tension without cracking under the strain. We must remember that, for all its resilience and its power to tolerate vast differences of tension without failing, there are nevertheless limits set to the resistance of the nervous system. Let us not forget that the difference between a gorilla and a primitive man is much smaller than that between a primitive man and a God-man. Just as a gorilla cannot be expected within a single lifetime to develop into a man because his physical constitution would be incapable of bridging the gap, so to an even lesser degree can a primitive man, or an average man who has just been 'awakened', be expected in a single lifetime to become a fully conscious and spiritualized God-man. The resilience of his nerves would not be adequate to the purpose.

But if one could tell a gorilla how he could *consciously* develop his under-developed brain centres by constant practice, and if he really did practise, and tried to exercise and learn the letters, figures and other things which were quite new to him, he would attain human status much more quickly, although not in his present gorilla life. Let us be quite clear about this: the gorilla could not develop and change the shape of his head, and hence his brain, to the extent that he became a man, but he could *exploit to the utmost the possibilities of his gorillahood*, and he would then take with him into the next life a much more developed body and a nervous system to match. This he would continue to exercise consciously until he had developed it to the limits of its potentialities. In this way he might in two or three lives become a human being, albeit a primitive one, but at a very much faster rate than if he were to pursue the simple path of natural development over several thousand years. The gorilla does not understand this conscious development – nor does primitive man – and so they develop in accordance with the laws of Nature. Eternity is long enough.

The man, however, who has grown out of the restricted consciousness of average being and is already sufficiently awakened not to be at his ease at his low level of development for the very reason that he already feels much greater potentialities astir in him, is accessible to instruction. It is possible to discuss with him how and by what means he can develop more rapidly and to a higher level than if he were to wait simply on the natural path until the resistance of his nerves had been automatically enhanced by the daily struggles of life. In this way, then, he will gradually be enabled by his increasingly resilient nerves to experience higher states of consciousness and to tolerate them without detriment to his health. Our book, therefore, is addressed to people who already realize that their rate of development can be speeded up by conscious exercises of the mind and body and who not only understand this but are also impelled by an ever-growing inner desire to take the trouble to exercise and consciously develop themselves. Admittedly there is one thing we must never forget and that is that, however great our determination to make progress, we can only advance as far as the potentialities of our body and our nervous system allow when realized to their extreme. We must not expect to reach the level of a God-man in a short time. We must rest content if we can realize the *highest potentialities inherent in our body* and our being in this life. And so it is also worth exercising because no human limits can be foreseen to this 'highest potentiality'. We normally have no idea of what a man is capable of bearing and enduring. Only in the dreadful trials brought by war or natural catastrophe do the unsuspected capacities and the unimaginable resistance of man become apparent. These capacities and the resilience of the body are, of course, dependent on the unknown power of the spiritual forces present. It follows therefore that we must not form any preconceptions of the limit of our potentialities – on the path of Yoga or elsewhere – or of the level which we can or cannot attain, for it is in the nature of things that we cannot know these in advance. Let us not worry ourselves about the precise rung of Jacob's ladder we have prospects of attaining in this life. Let us leave that to God. We should exercise with absolute trust and faith in God so as to lose no time but to progress as quickly as possible. In any case we shall take with us at the moment of our deaths the stage of development we have attained in this life, and in our next life we shall begin with this highest stage as the lowest stage of our new incarnation. None of our efforts will be wasted!

We shall not go into the pathology of sex here. Those who are of such a disposition will understand their condition better if they take the contents of this book properly to heart and also find the way to liberation. Here we shall confine our remarks to the stages through which one must gradually pass from sexual pathology to health and from health to the supreme and divinely spiritual level, and how and whence the strength for this purpose may be derived.

We want to show the connections between the path of Yoga – the way of expanding consciousness – and this supremely important, natural and healthy, but quickened progress in the control of sexual energy, and place the key to the true and healthy conversion and spiritualization of vitalizing sexual energy in the hands of the many practitioners of Yoga who come to our Yoga school and also those who wish to practise Yoga successfully at home.

A dear old friend, who was nevertheless still in possession of his youthful vigour, once told me this story. He went for a walk with a good friend, who was much older than himself. On their walk his friend told him that although he had lost his virile powers he still enjoyed life to the full since the pleasures of the mind were infinitely great. He read great books, often went to the theatre and opera, travelled widely, played golf and so forth. My friend listened to him for a time and then said: 'My dear friend, don't go on about the delights of your life, for you won't succeed in making me want to be impotent!'

Now it is not the intention of this book to make anyone 'want to be impotent'. Far from it! Indeed it sets out to do the very opposite: to show the practitioner of Yoga *the way that leads to the source of the very highest potency*. And if along this path one reaches the final goal, the final goal of all humanity, then at the same time one attains spiritual mastery over all the powers which are always potentially present in the great divine self of man and of all living creatures. And once this spiritual mastery has been attained, it is never lost again, not even as the body grows old, for the divine-creative powers are not derived from the body but *create* the body. And anyone who has recognized and felt them in himself and has learnt to use them as a key, has obtained conscious control over his body.

The source of supreme potency is God.

And so what this book sets out to do is to show the shortest way to God!

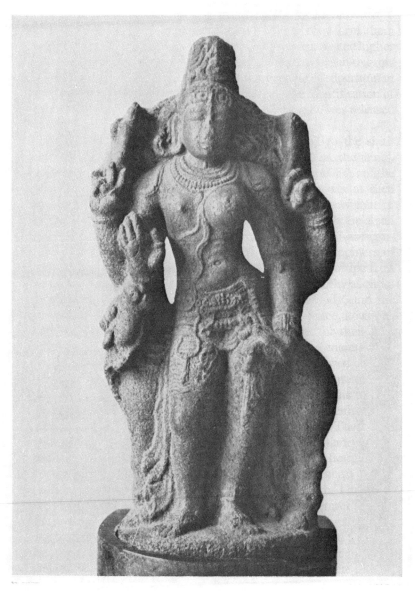

In GOD the two poles rest within each other in perfect unity and harmony, in absolute equilibrium. Indian philosophy of religion depicts this truth in the figure of the god Shiva, who unites the two sexes within himself. (Reproduction by courtesy of the Rietberg Museum, Zürich.)

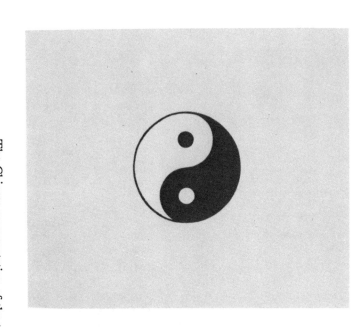

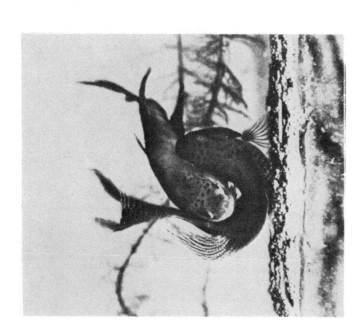

The Chinese representation of the two poles of creation in their primal state. They are called Yin and Yang, the positive pole and the negative pole, the giving and the receiving, the power and the resistance. They rest in the primal state, in GOD, in perfect equilibrium and absolute harmony within each other. Physical, sexual union is an imitation and reflection of this divine unity.

# Chapter 2

# Recognition and Being are One

It has been the trend of human development for us to work less and less while allowing external forms of energy, like light, heat, electricity, magnetism, radio-activity or nuclear energy to do our work for us more and more. We take this for granted. These kinds of energy we use every day and life is hardly imaginable without them. But if we wish to know what they really are, what comprises their true substance, and study the books of the greatest contemporary scientists, we come to the conclusion that we can only observe and know these various forms of energy, as indeed all things, from outside. We can only describe the *behaviour* of substances which have been heated, electrified, magnetized, radio-activated or ionized. But we do not and cannot ever know the real and true nature of this energy or of anything else. It is impossible for us because we ourselves *are* not this energy or any of the things of this world. That is to say, our state of being is not identical with that of all these things.

Each thing could alone know and tell what it essentially is, whether it is a form of energy or a living creature such as a cat or dog, for only forms of energy or a cat or a dog could know and tell what a form of energy, a cat or a dog is, simply because they are what they are, but only if they could speak, and what is paramount, *if they were conscious in themselves!*

But that is impossible. Impossible, because everything that has been and will be created is naturally what it is – the different forms of energy, the elements, plants, animals and finally man in his unconscious state – all these are what they are, yet they do not know of themselves what they are, because they are not conscious in themselves.

Man alone is capable of attaining complete self-knowledge,

complete self-awareness, and only the awakened man, who has become completely conscious in his true being, with *not one particle of the latter remaining unconscious*, only he knows of himself what he is. And when a man has attained this perfect state of self-awareness he will be in a position to know of *a single force of energy in the entire creation* – but here again he experiences *the essential nature of this energy* not from without, but from within, in a state of being. *And this is his own vitality in all its manifestations, from the lowest materialized form, known as sexual energy, to its highest form, the divine creative power, for the true nature of this energy is simultaneously his own true nature : he is it itself!* In the first person: *I am it!*

The attainment of this knowledge is the final goal of his path! For man also began his career as an unconscious living creature, and at the lowest level of his humanity he has only an outward-looking consciousness, like an animal. And so long as his self-awareness has not awakened and after long development, perhaps over eons, become one in a state of being with his own self, in its entirety, man too cannot – and does not – know what his true being is, what he is in reality. And in this unconscious condition it is as impossible for him to know what he is as to know what electricity, radio-activity, nuclear energy or other forms of energy are, and what the essence of the energy is that gave him his own life and that enables him to pass on life, that is to say, he does not know what sexual energy is.

In the First Epistle to the Corinthians, Paul the Apostle clearly expresses the truth that each thing can itself alone know what it is, and nothing else, since it can only be in a state of being with itself:

But God hath revealed them unto us by his Spirit: for the Spirit searcheth all things, yea, the deep things of God. For what man knoweth the things of a man, save the spirit of man which is in him? even so the things of God knoweth no man, but the Spirit of God. Now we have received not the spirit of the world, but the spirit which is God; that we might know the things that are freely given to us of God. Which things also we speak, not in the words which man's wisdom teacheth, but which the Holy Ghost teacheth: comparing spiritual things with spiritual. But the natural man receiveth not the things of the

Spirit of God: for they are foolishness unto him: neither can he know them, because they are spiritually discerned. But he that is spiritual judgeth all things, yet he himself is judged of no man. (I Cor. 2:10–15.)

In modern language we might formulate it thus: If we ourselves were not human, we could not know the nature of a human being. If we did not embrace the Spirit of God, we could not even know that there is a God, or what God is. But we have received the Spirit of God and have become conscious in it; therefore we have knowledge of divine things. The unconscious man – or as Paul calls him: 'the natural man', does not yet know what lies behind his consciousness, hence he regards spiritual truths as foolishness. The man who has attained consciousness knows, however, that as a human being he embraces the Spirit of God, and thus he stands above all earthly, worldly things.

Man at the first and lowest level of his humanity is still nothing more than an animal plus reason. He confuses his 'SELF' with his consciousness. He believes that in saying 'I' he has designated his whole SELF. In fact he has only designated with the word 'I' that small personal part of his SELF which has already become conscious in himself. He does not know the unconscious part of his Self, therefore he does not recognize it or even suspect its existence. His unconscious assumes the guise of external beings; this is how concepts such as 'devil' and 'angel' have arisen. At this low level he does not know that these fictive beings are in reality also powers from his own unconscious, that is that they are *himself*. He still has no idea whatsoever that there exists behind his primitive consciousness, although for the time being inaccessible to him, an infinitely greater part of his SELF in a totally unconscious state. How could he then know the nature of his *whole* true being? How could he know that God himself dwells within him, that he is in reality a divine being, if he knows neither God nor his true Self, nor that this true Self *is* God!

People who have attained complete consciousness in their total Self – in God, who have attained universal consciousness, were, and still are, very rare on earth. Nevertheless, the sole aim of all our lives, of our reincarnations, is to attain this complete consciousness, and to become one in a monistic state of being with the Creator who rests in the profound depths of our souls, as I AM!

But how can unconscious animal man become aware and attain this goal if he is ignorant of it? Born the first time as a human being on the lowest rung of the great Jacob's ladder of consciousness, how can he ascend step by step from this state, elevate himself to divine self-awareness, to the perfect fulfilment and resurrection, if he is unaware of the existence of this goal and of his own ability to attain it? What helps him, what impels him suddenly to direct his outward-looking consciousness inwards for the first time, to become 'converted', and to rise from the first awakening, from the first faint glimmer of self-awareness to universal consciousness, to the divine and radiant celestial being which is inherent within him, and to attain release, liberation and resurrection?

What urges him to do this, and to raise himself, is none other than his own sexual energy!

This gigantic energy is latent in every living creature. It first helps a human being through his parents to be born into matter, into a body, and when he has reached physical maturity it gives him the ability to endow further beings with a body. The unconscious man, however, still does not realize that this very energy not only enables him to beget children, but also that it is the only force, the impulse which helps, indeed compels him to raise his consciousness stage by stage to the divine state of self-awareness. Sexual energy forces human consciousness in an upward direction and drives it ever higher. It goes without saying that, until he reaches the highest stage of self-awareness and self-realization, a human being cannot know that as such he can become familiar only with this energy, and this alone, in its true being. But he can, and indeed will, make this energy conscious in himself, for it is his true being, *it is himself.*

*Sexual energy helps man to rise above sexual energy!* Has this not been decreed with infinite wisdom?

If we ever experience this truth ourselves, then we can understand why the initiated used the scorpion as the symbol of sexual energy. The scorpion is the agent of its own destruction, and in the same way sexual power destroys itself because it compels the unconscious man and aids the conscious man to transform sexual energy into higher energies and to come to self-awareness in this energy – *to be this very energy!* But it is then no longer sexual energy; it has destroyed itself as such.

Let us attempt to penetrate the mystery of sexual energy that we might recognize it in ourselves and obtain mastery over it. How can this be done? We shall answer this question in the following chapters.

# Chapter 3

# The Creative Primal Serpent

The Gospel according to St John opens with following words:

In the beginning was the Word and the Word was with God, and the Word was God. The same was in the beginning with God. All things were made by him; and without him was not any thing made that was made. In him was life; and the life was the light of men. And the light shineth in darkness; and the darkness comprehended it not.

How admirably do these few words elucidate the mystery of the creation!

But we could only properly understand and appreciate these words if we could read the Bible in the Greek original. The translation is, alas, not always a correct one. The English language lacks the words for an exact rendering of the Greek text. There is no word which means the same as the Greek word *logos*, and so Luther translated *logos* with 'word', which completely fails to render the meaning of *logos*. It would have been better to take 'verb' because it expresses more adequately the birth of the first motion, the first stirring of creation. In Greek, *logos* means the creative principle, the power of God, the instrument of God which executes his will and animates the creation, as, for instance, a man's hand, which is at the same time himself and his instrument, which is *active*. When *logos* was still in its latent primal state, before anything, even before God's very first revelation, the creation of vowels and letters, 'the word' which is composed of letters likewise could not have existed. That is an essentially later phase of creation. And apart from this there is an added difficulty in understanding this text correctly. Each individual has his own interpretation of many of the words according to his lower or higher level of consciousness. The word

'God' means something different to each person. It is true, and can be verified in the Greek original, that God created man 'on' the mould of his image just as the glove is drawn over the hand, and he continues to do so today; it is equally true that man reciprocates this by creating God in his own human image. Moreover, the words used in Luther's time are no longer suitable to express certain things. If we then try to render the meaning of these sentences according to the *Greek original* with modern words, it would run something like this: In the beginning was *logos*, the will that brings forth the deed, the power that animates and realizes creation, still with God in a latent condition, as God's potency. God was and is this power himself. Essentially, God and his creative principle, his creative power, are one and the same thing. All things were created by God through *logos*. God is being, is life itself, and everything that exists can only do so because the creative principle, the creative aspect of God, namely, *logos*, creates, animates and sustains it. God, eternal being, life, moulded man too – according to the original text – *on* himself, *on* his own image. Therefore the true Self, the very essence of man is God himself. But man *in his unconscious condition* is still in darkness and does not comprehend God's light within himself. He is unaware and has no inkling that God, that is, his quintessential Self, dwells in his unconscious.

Life is therefore the creative power, *logos*, and everything that was created was created by *logos*. Everything from the rarest spirit to matter was and is created, animated and sustained by *logos*. But at the seventh and very highest level is the spirit of God, God himself in a perfectly balanced state of repose. From here, God, as his own creative principle – for *logos is* God himself – creates the entire scale of creation. From infinite space, from every point of the universe, from everywhere, life flows. At first purely spiritual forms of energy of the highest frequencies arise and take effect, then the frequencies gradually slow down, the waves become longer, and the forms of manifestation continue acquiring density and substance till the lowest level is reached, that of the so-called 'dead' matter, which is, however, not dead, for we know that matter is simply another form of energy. In the atom of matter, just as in the solar and astronomical systems, God's creative power circulates, life circulates. It is in every rung of Jacob's ladder which reaches from heaven, from the kingdom of God, down to the material world, to earth.

We human beings bear all forms of creative energy within us. We are the microcosm in the macrocosm. Our spirit, our true Self, is God, as Paul has already stated. Then *logos*, the creative power of the Self, descends deeper into us as in the universe, forms our ideas, creates the emotional and spiritual levels and finally the necessary resistance to these, the bearer of all higher forms of energy, our physical body. Just as *logos*, beyond man, and at all levels of creation, manifests and creates *itself* as different forms of energy, so do we human beings bear the whole Jacob's ladder of *logos*-manifestations, that is, entire creation as the various aspects of our own Self. And as *logos* is active at each level of creation in the macrocosm, so man emits and manifests in his microcosm at each level of his being, through the organs corresponding to the various frequencies of the creative power, the outward forms of the same divine, creative energy, that is to say, of our own Self.

If we draw the human spine with the brain and its extension the spinal cord, we observe the form of a serpent. This serpent is by the same token the image of the manifestation form of the *logos* in the macrocosm, and in man, the microcosm. It is also the image of the resistance to the *logos*, of its locus in man: the spinal cord. This 'spinal serpent' created from the finest ethereal matter is the bearer of the divine creative power, of our own life. The power emanates with gradually increasing frequencies from seven spiritual centres, by way of suitable organs which sustain the creative power as resistance.

In Ancient Egypt the initiated wore a band of gold on their headdress, which symbolized a serpent with erect head. To be 'initiated' meant that a man had become conscious at all seven levels of self-revelation or self-awareness, and therefore in the *logos*-serpent as a whole. There was no longer an unconscious element and so he was a man who had attained universal consciousness.

The erect Aesculapian serpent drinking the elixir of life from a shallow goblet also represents the creative life-force serpent in the human spine. It is the absolute wholeness, therefore health, and consequently also has the power to heal all diseases – that is to say, all forms of degeneration.

We find the same 'serpent' in India, there known as 'Kundalini'. As long as man remains unconscious with his higher nerve centres still in a latent condition, the serpent rests coiled up in the lowest centre of energy which has its seat in the terminal vertebra, the coccyx; that is, in the negative pole of vital tension! As man gradually becomes conscious and his energy centres are activated in the process, the Kundalini serpent slowly uncoils itself and stretches up and up, lays hold of and animates each succeeding nerve centre, and ascends to the very highest centre, which has its seat in the uppermost part of the head, in the skull. There it unites with the positive pole which lies in the seventh energy centre. Then it stands as erect as the Aesculapian serpent.

The philosophy of Yoga lays great stress on the difference between the vital current and the resistance, namely the physical organs and nerve centres by which the current is borne. Creative power, the vital current, forms seven energy centres in man's being, and each energy centre, known in the terminology of Yoga as *chakra*, has the effect of a transformer which transforms the divine creative power to a lower tension corresponding to the next centre of manifestation. Thus, proceeding from the uppermost centre, creative power is transformed six times and there are as a result seven energy centres, seven *chakras*.

Since we human beings have become familiar with this energy from the earthly, material level, we start counting the energy focuses, which are at the same time the levels of manifestation, from the bottom upwards. The Yoga terms for these seven centres are Sanskrit words as follows:

The first and lowest *chakra* is called: Muladhara (*Mula* means 'marrow'); its seat is in the negative pole, which rests in the coccyx in a latent condition.

Second *chakra*: Svadisthana; its seat is in the nerve plexus above the genital organs.

Third *chakra*: Manipura; its seat is in the solar plexus.

Fourth *chakra*: Anahata; its seat is in the nerve centre of the heart.

Fifth *chakra*: Vishuddha; its seat is in the nerve centre of the thyroid gland.

Sixth *chakra*: Adjna; its seat is in the centre of the forehead, between the eyebrows.

Seventh *chakra*: Sahasrara; its seat is in the uppermost part of the skull, which is also the seat of the positive pole. Through the activation of this brain centre man attains divine all-consciousness.

In the Bible, day or light means: *consciousness*. Night or darkness means: *unconsciousness*. According to this metaphor, as Moses the great initiate says in the Bible, God creates every 'day' at all levels of consciousness with the vibrations pertaining to the levels, but at the seventh level of consciousness, on the seventh 'day', he does not create, but rests in himself. In this state there is no tension from which a creation could be evolved, because the two poles, the positive one and the negative one, are resting reconciled in one another in perfect balance and absolute oneness. Man can only experience this in a state of ecstasy as pure consciousness, otherwise it would mean physical death.

In the works of some Western scholars we read that the Indian yogi in the ecstatic Samadhi is unconscious. That is a great error! The opposite is true: he is in the state of *complete consciousness*, therefore of *universal consciousness*. He appears to be unconscious from outside only because he has no physical consciousness. Whoever has himself experienced the Samadhi state will know that, during it, the yogi is completely *conscious* and fully *awake*.

From this we may observe that there is only one truth and that the core of every religion is this sole truth. St Francis of Assisi, St Theresa and other great saints experienced the divine presence in an ecstatic state just as the Indian yogis in Asia have experienced it as 'Samadhi' and are still doing so.

We human beings experience these various levels of the *logos* – manifestations and various frequencies as various states of consciousness. Accordingly, we give them various names.

The energy form of divine power, which links mind and matter at the first level in the lowest centre, we experience in our conscious mind as the instinct for the preservation of the species, as sexual, physical urge and desire, and in fulfilment as purely physical gratification. This we call *sexual energy*.

At the second level we experience it as the manifestation of the self-preservation instinct, as metabolism; in our conscious mind as hunger and thirst, and in fulfilment as repletion.

At the third level divine power emanates as will-power and we experience it in our conscious mind as the urge towards volition.

At the fourth level divine power prevails through the heart centre, the feelings and emotions. In our conscious mind we experience it as sensibility, as feelings; we experience the whole scale between hate and personal love which are mirror images.

At the fifth level divine power manifests itself as our concept of time and space. Its instrument is the thyroid gland which connects us with the finite world; it links us with time and provides our *time rhythm*. This centre determines the fast or slow tempo of our thoughts and movements, whether we find a period of time long or short, whether we are always in haste or take things at an easy pace. Consequently this centre exercises a decisive influence on the tempo of our life-rhythm, and thus on the temporal duration of our life.

At the sixth level the *logos*-energy manifests itself as intuition. It flashes into our conscious mind the lightning, as it were, of spiritual light, which provides us with new ideas and insights. As a state of consciousness we experience this intuition as all-pervading spiritual light, spiritual meditation and, identical with this, as all-embracing universal love. We feel a sense of oneness with the whole universe, we understand the language of Nature and the symbolic content of every line and form.

At the seventh and highest level, through the centre in the uppermost part of the skull, we experience divine creative power as a purely spiritual state of being; this appears in our conscious mind as the profoundest self-knowledge, as supreme *'individual consciousness'* which we experience in ourselves as 'I AM THAT I AM'. Here there are no longer unconscious feelings or thoughts, no longer outward-looking perceptions. I am no longer happy and content, because '*I am*' these things, all feelings, all thoughts, the radiant light of consciousness – '*I myself am*' happiness, '*I myself am*' bliss and peace! *I am a radiant, all-embracing, all-penetrating self-awareness.*

During excavations in Mexico symbolic representations of God were found. They give apt and clear illustration of this truth and of these various forms of divine manifestation at the different levels of creation. At the base there is a serpent or sometimes a dragon, that is sexual energy: Kundalini. On it stands a man's figure which symbolizes the body – sustaining, emotional, mental and intuitive manifestations, and at the very top, above the man, is a radiant face, the face of God, the symbol of pure spiritual, divine self-awareness: God! How could one have better depicted the truth of the various manifestation forms of one and the same deity?

Man alone is capable of attaining consciousness at all levels of creation and of embracing all the manifestation levels in a divine universal consciousness. This is because man alone has in his body the organs corresponding to the various forms of creative energy. These organs are able to bear, as the matching resistance, the different vibrations and frequencies of the various forms in which the universal, creative energy is manifested. Just as the organs are suited to receive these vibrations and frequencies from the universe, so, on the other hand, are they also capable of emitting these creating energies. These organs are the most important nerve and brain centres which transmit the vibrations of the various creative energy forms to the corresponding glands closely linked to the centres in which the transformation takes place. In the man who is at the lowest level of his humanity the majority of these nerve and brain centres are still in a dormant condition. His degree of consciousness is accordingly low and primitive. The path of his development lies in mastering and activating each succeeding centre until all the nerve and brain centres have been activated and man has made the whole scale of creation, *including the Creator*, conscious in himself.

The fuel with which man can heat and activate his latent nerve and brain centres, somewhat like a radio valve, is the sexual energy which he bears in his body. As long as man remains at a low level of consciousness he is not master of his sexual energy, but rather its servant. He is still completely its slave and at its mercy. Therefore he never even suspects that this energy embodies a secret, that his own sexual energy can open the door to spiritual power, that with the help of this energy he can attain consciousness in his divine Self and in God and thence acquire immortality, ascendancy over matter and over the whole of Nature. Through this he has found the secret key to the philosopher's stone, he has become a white magician.

The medieval alchemists, the Rosicrucians, who were great initiates, repeatedly point out in their curious writings, in which the naked truth is always avoided, that the substance from which the philosopher's stone can be made is very easily found and all human beings are in possession of it. They wished to protect their knowledge from the vulgar who even then would have turned everything to mischief and out of sheer ignorance abused the secret of sexual energy for depraved perversions. At the same time, however, they wished to pass on the key to this secret only to such people as were sufficiently mature not to abuse it. They wished to direct men of intelligence to the right path *where* they should look for the secret in the hope that some would find it. It is quite clear from their writings that the substance for the philosopher's stone *is to be found in man himself.* Merely this harmless clue led to dreadful cruelties. We know from medieval court records that lords who wanted to make the philosopher's stone regarded human blood as the secret substance, for they interpreted the Rosicrucian writings to mean that the stone was to be formed out of a human being. Thus with unbelievable cruelty they slaughtered their serfs wholesale in order to obtain the substance from their bodies. In their ignorance these lords, like the Apostle Paul's 'natural men', the unaware, ignorant 'dead' people, never realized that the matter was much simpler than they thought. They should only have remembered that the source through which all earthly life is transmitted is sexual energy. The source of life, the famous elixir of the Rosicrucians, is therefore something we bear within us! From this source flows a current, life itself, 'which is fire, but flows like water'. What better definition could they have found of the kind of energy that flows like electricity or water into our nervous system, yet is not water but fire; therefore as literally stated in the Rosicrucian writings, 'a fiery water, the watery fire' is 'a current of fire, which flows like water'. The ignorant man uses this 'individual source', usually his sexual, vital energy, in the pursuit of erotic pleasures and without desire to procreate. He does not realize that if he were not to expend the vital current which flows from his 'individual source', but to preserve it for his own body and to use the life-source for himself, he could kindle and activate his higher energy centres, the *chakras*, and thereby obtain mastery over them. If he were to use the vital current for his own body, as the will demands, he could then endow his body with new life, regenerate it and even attain the immortality of the cells known to the Rosicrucians as transmutation. Through the higher spiritual centres he could creatively use sexual energy, converted into creative spiritual power, to serve himself and at the same time share in the labour of spiritualizing our world. In order to possess himself of this secret, it is *absolutely essential that a man has a superior morality and attitude to life!* And since these are exceedingly rare, the 'alchemists', the Rosicrucians and other initiates spoke only in symbols or not at all.

Today, in contrast to that age, we have reached the stage where these things must be discussed in order to awaken man's morality. And this not for reasons of sentimental religiosity, but rather for general, human ones, since God so created the spiritual constitution of man that if he resists the inner moral laws inherent in all men he will inevitably bring misery, despair and spiritual darkness upon himself. Men have misunderstood and misinterpreted certain truths discovered by great psychiatrists. And, what is worse, confused by the errors which semi-ignorant charlatans disseminate, they abuse their sexual energy by treating it more and more as a merely physical phenomenon and employing it almost exclusively for erotic pleasures. This attitude is fraught with such great danger that we wish to try and arouse the attention of those seekers and in particular of the young people led astray by the erroneous interpretation of 'repression', 'liberation from spiritual and physical inhibitions' and of 'freedom from inhibition'. We do this even though we know for certain that many people will again use the secret of sexual energy for degenerate perversions. It must be said quite frankly that sexual energy can be used for much higher purposes than merely relieving with erotic experience the boredom arising from one's own infinite emptiness. Sexual energy is divine creative power itself. It can be used for heaven or hell. But if it is used for hellish purposes it strikes back and plunges its abuser inexorably into hell.

Perhaps there will be some among the many misled young people and adults who will lend an ear and, perhaps at first out of sheer curiosity, risk an experiment for at least a certain time. In the course of these experiments they will garner such profound experiences that they will once and for all set foot on the path of truth and never again swerve from it. And there will certainly also be many people, indeed there are already, who will undertake this labour out of a true sense of longing for God. If only a few are thus led to the right path, this book will have fulfilled its purpose.

In order to conduct the experiments properly and to form any idea at all of what they are about, we must first make ourselves familiar with a few things and turn them over in our minds. For this book also sets out to show the way of tried and proven practice. Christ prophesies in the Bible that a time will come when the mysteries of truth will be proclaimed upon the housetops. There are a number of striking indications that this time has come. The point has been reached where the truth about sexual energy must be disclosed. What men make of it depends on their moral maturity. After all, nuclear energy can be used for better purposes than the making of weapons man plans to use for his own annihilation! In the same way it is possible to use sexual energy for heaven or hell since it is the divine creative power or *logos*, the essence of man himself. When man has taken hold of spiritual, magical power and thus attained supremacy, it rests with himself whether he becomes a black or a white magician!

# Chapter 4

# Sexual Energy in its False and True Light

In Revelation (5:6) we read how *logos* in the guise of a Lamb with seven horns and seven eyes sets out to embody itself in matter, to animate and spiritualize it and trace it back to God:

> ... and in the midst of the elders, stood a Lamb as it had been slain [in matter, in the body, the spirit feels as if it had been slain]; having seven horns and seven eyes, which are the seven Spirits of God sent forth into all the earth.

And: 'Behold the Lamb of God, which taketh away the sin of the world.' (St John 1:29.) 'Taking away the sin of the world' means for the spirit to assume the burden of the attributes of matter. For the body, which is matter, the attributes of matter are not sin; for the spirit, they are. The attributes, namely the laws of matter, are diametrically opposed to those of the spirit. In his Epistle to the Galatians (5:17–18) Paul says:

> For the flesh lusteth against the Spirit and the Spirit against the flesh: and these are contrary the one to the other: so that ye cannot do the things that ye would. But if ye be led of the Spirit, ye are not under the law [of the flesh, of matter].

The laws of matter are contraction, cooling, stiffening, hardening and solidification. The laws of the spirit are fire, warmth, heat, expansion and radiation. Therefore it is sinful for the spirit to manifest the attributes of matter. And in the same way it is sinful for matter to manifest the attributes of the spirit. The Lamb of God is spirit, and if it embodies itself in matter it must subject itself to the laws of matter and accept the attributes of matter, which for the Lamb are sin. Only in this way can *logos* spiritualize matter and trace it back to God.

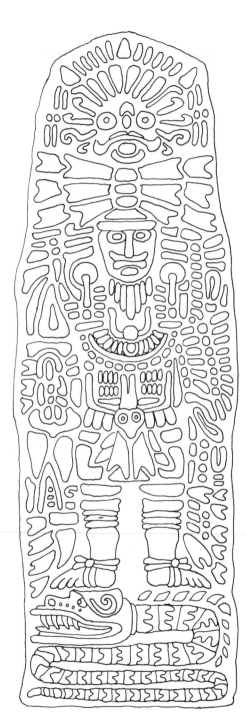

Representation of God in Ancient Mexico: at the base is a serpent, symbolizing sexual energy; on it stands a man's figure which symbolizes the body-sustaining, emotional, mental and intuitive manifestations; at the very top is the incorporeal, pure spiritual and radiant self-awareness: GOD.

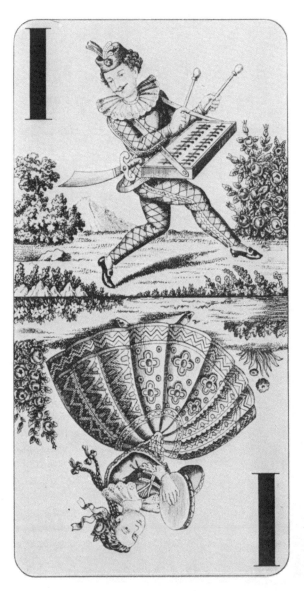

The first and lowest tarot card represents the human beings who are still 'dead', still unconscious in spirit and who lead a purely physical existence. They are at first still separate human beings – 'man' and 'woman' – and think only in terms of sex. These are the tiny marionettes, the 'homunculi', which dance round on the palm of the great sexless Ego as their earthly role desires.

The creative principle, *logos*, the Lamb of God, says of itself in another passage of the Bible: '*I am* the way, the truth, and the life: no man cometh unto the Father, but by *me*.' (St John 14:6.) Thus the life that *I* myself *am*, in the very words of the *logos*, is itself the path by which we come to the Father. For this purpose life first embodied itself in matter, out of it formed a suitable shell, a body, and built into this body organs capable of begetting ever further bodies. The divine current of life flows uninterruptedly through these bodies, forming ever new shells, which become ever more able to bear and to manifest the vibrations of the spirit as resistance. And while the material, living and yet unconscious shell, the person, lives his shadowy existence, he is being wrought, indeed tormented, out of his unconscious mind by life, which in its materialized form is sexual energy, in order that his consciousness may be roused. In the individual, still unconscious part of his material being, primitive man's higher Self, *logos*, constantly impels him by means of sexual energy to become conscious in himself, in his material body, and to come to know the essence of his deepest being, God, that is to say, *to attain self-knowledge*. As long as man remains unconscious, he experiences God within himself as sexual desire. When he has become conscious, he experiences God as his own *Self*, as his own true being, as *I am*! – God is for man the absolute *state of self-awareness*.

In this way life, the eternal being, God, helps *itself* to grow more conscious in matter, in the body, till such time as the greatest miracle has been wrought: one and the same divine self-awareness embraces the opposing spiritual and material laws, matter is spiritualized, and in this spiritualized body the creative principle, *logos*, the Lamb of God which died into matter at birth, is at last resurrected after eons of development, and has again become itself, God. The Lamb and his wife, *logos* and the consciousness of the physical being have become *one*. The heavenly, mystical marriage has been performed!

Misunderstanding of the Scriptures and incorrect religious instruction have led Western man to regard the procreation of ever-new generations, without which life would cease, and the physical enjoyment and sensation of pleasure associated with this, as the work of the Devil. He has allowed the concept of 'original sin' to be imprinted in his mind, and indeed to this very day regards the physical organs requisite to procreation as sinful and obscene. How admirably pure and divine is on the other hand the conception of some ancient and contemporary Asian peoples who regard the male genital organ, the Lingam, as sacred, and worship it as the outward material form of the divine, since its very purpose is to manifest and propagate the supreme: life, eternal being, God, through matter, through the body. It is naïve to a degree to suppose that the Orientals' worship of the Lingam involves worship of the merely physical male organ. Do they still believe in the West that antiquity and the Orientals who have achieved the supreme culture were and are so foolish as to worship a specific *member of the body*? The Orientals do not and have never worshipped matter or the body as such, but rather *the godhead manifesting itself* through the material form! Their entire philosophy of religion, their absolute disparagement of the physical clearly show this exalted mentality. Similarly, Western man is quite misled in seeing no more than mere pornography in the noble representations of the sexual act which adorn the majestic sun-god temples in Konarak, Bubaneshvar and other Indian temples. The inspired Indians who created these breathtaking, magnificent works of art did not regard the sexual act as obscene but as the imitation of the primal state of God, as the image of life, in which the two poles rest within each other and in which a new life, a new incarnation is made possible. They regarded the sexual act as the very deity which manifests itself through matter, separated into two halves, into two sexes but also reunited through the sexes to propagate earthly life in matter, so that the great aim may be achieved and realized, *to spiritualize matter, to attain divine self-awareness in matter, to experience the resurrection of human consciousness in God!*

It is a mystery how the white race has come to regard the sexual act which has given life to us and to our children as obscene and unmentionable. If it is something to be ashamed of why do the people who hold such views continue to perform it? And why then did God so create the world, according to these people, that this wicked act is absolutely necessary for the procreation of living creatures?

What a vast difference there is between the Eastern and the Western conceptions. On the one hand the Lingam is regarded as the embodiment of the forces of life and in it the divine is worshipped in order to beget children; on the other hand, the genital organ has been severed from the perfect, classical representations of Greek and Roman gods and the damaged parts covered with a vine or fig-leaf. (It is as if one had wished to attract even more attention to them.) Men who act in such a way betray their own sexual pathology. Instead of regarding the sexual act as an exalted fulfilment of the desire for oneness, for love, as a life-giving act in imitation of God, affording real contentment and happiness, they regard it as a brutish end in itself, good only for wanton and depraved sensual enjoyment, which has nothing whatever to do with love and true happiness. If these people thought differently, they would have no reason to cover up the genital organs as something obscene. By their own primitive mentality *they* cast the shadow of obscenity over the genital organs. These people drag the divine down into their own impurity. The fault lies, however, not in the divine, vitalizing force and sexual act, but in the attitude of those who so pervert these things that they have real cause to be ashamed. No wonder that the time had to come when the pendulum swung from prudery in the other direction. As a result there are today many pathological people who, on the one hand, attach excessive importance to sexuality by seeking a sexual cause for *every* mental disorder and, on the other hand, make light of sexual energy by provoking uninhibited sexual intercourse at every opportunity. As if sexual union were a cigarette to be smoked and then thrown away and forgotten! These people do not know that sexual energy is a manifestation of the *being of man* himself, and that there can be no sexual intercourse *without* conscious or unconscious *self-surrender*. The partner, whether male or female, is not an object to be used and discarded, but is a living creature and also has a human soul. This is true even of prostitutes! These misguided people try to satisfy their longing for happiness and mental stability by means of purely physical, sexual intercourse. People yearn for love, but not for purely physical gratification.

It is a dangerous error to seek love in soulless sexuality and to try to replace love by sexuality. It is natural enough for, say, women who are never given the slightest expression of love by their lifeless, uninteresting and uninterested 'dead' husbands to believe that the tokens of tenderness shown by a husband interested in his wife during the brief period of sexual excitement constitute love and therefore to want to have sexual intercourse with their husbands as often as they can. This is not because they are primarily interested in sexual intercourse as such, but because they long for 'a little bit of love'. If the husband fails them, and if an opportunity arises – which it nearly always does! – they then try to get love from *another* man and to experience sexuality to the full. In most cases they do not really do this out of physical frustration. The body desires sexual gratification far less often than one imagines! Men long for women to look up to them and admire them as the highest manifestation of God, as *man*. If a man does not get this recognition at home, he will certainly meet another woman who pays him the tribute of admiration and afterwards it usually looks as if he had only wanted sex. The man as well as the woman looks for 'love' from his or her lover but they are wrong to believe that this is received from this 'other' partner. They meet secretly and, because they always expect sexual intercourse, in a state of sexual excitement. And sexuality mimics love. It compels tenderness and embraces, it forces the lovers to hug one another, to allay one another's pain through the revelations of sexuality, as when true love is exchanged. What follows such experiences? Disappointments, a bitter after-taste, mutual accusations or bleak loneliness, and, in the case of women, usually a desperate feeling of exploitation and defilement. *Neither of the two gave true love but only expected to receive it, therefore neither received it!* Love can never be replaced by empty, purely physical sexuality! And humanity yearns, languishes for *love*! These countless poor young souls, who are still little more than children and who, largely because the 'civilized' way of life is no longer conducive to love, perhaps went short of love from their parents, give themselves up to sexual adventures and excesses because they are searching for *love*! The many soul-sick people, young or old, can be healed only by love and not by cheapening sexual intercourse or by wishing to free them from sexual inhibitions and persuading them to lead a dissolute, promiscuous and indiscriminate sex life. How many of these people, young and old, seek advice on how to regain their lost physical and spiritual purity after such irresponsible psychic treatment. And if one shows them only a little love and understanding, they return to life healed and ready to become useful members of society. We have not come across one of those people who suffered 'repression' or 'trauma' from the purity enjoined on them. By 'purity' is meant of course not only a continent love-life, but also a healthy one based on *love*.

After the swing to extreme, indiscriminate 'permissiveness' and false conceptions of sexual 'freedom', caused by 'repression' and 'trauma', let us try to settle the pendulum in the middle and come to a normal conception of sexuality.

We should follow the example of great initiates who do not regard sexual energy as a malignant force but understand its secret and know that it is the sole means by which we human beings can attain the final goal – God. Here again the infinite wisdom with which entire creation is decreed reveals itself. Just as our ignorance alone brings us knowledge,[1] so it is sexual energy alone which brings us liberation from itself, from sexual energy. Sexual energy frees us from the very sexual desires to which it gives rise again and again and leads us from mortality, from death, to redemption, resurrection, to LIFE.

The medieval alchemists, the Rosicrucians, depicted this process of development very cleverly: the sage makes the philosopher's stone by placing his tree of life in a washing-trough filled with the elixir of life. This is constantly heated by the fire of the dragon, sexual energy, to make the tree blossom.

Let us not therefore despise sexuality or regard it as the malignant force which reduces man to an animal, nor let us *make* of it such a force.

Let us look upon sexual energy as the key which opens the door for us between spirit and the world of matter, from the higher to the lower but also from the lower to the higher. Let us regard it, then, as the divine impetus which enables us to create further generations, to propagate life from above downwards in the body but also to transform man upwards out of his ferity into a spiritual man and to help to conquer death. We must be grateful that sexual energy, used properly, gives us so much happiness on both paths. On the downward path it is brief and transient, on the upward path it is eternal happiness.

Let us use its fire to make our tree of life flourish and blossom. Let us remember: primitive man is still at the lowest level of his consciousness. In his animal egoism he lives within himself completely isolated and immured; his heart is still dead and he still has

[1] cf. Elisabeth Haich: *Ein paar Worte über Magie*.

no inkling of the meaning of love. Sexual energy, that elemental fire, is alone able to warm his dead heart for the first time. And even if during the brief spell of sexual excitement he can experience and express only an inkling of love, it is notwithstanding the first glimmer of divine love. Through sexuality he first becomes acquainted with the happiness derived from giving. And although his dawning love is still no more than an animal desire, a passion, his excitement is, even if only quite unconsciously and briefly, already an urge towards oneness, towards love! Even if at first he experiences this urge towards love only in the body and hence can only look for *physical* gratification, it is nevertheless the first reflection of spiritual oneness in the great Self, which man is unconsciously seeking and which, after long development, perhaps over eons, he will find because he is destined to do so. Sexual energy causes us inner unrest which never allows us to stand still. It continually spurs us on and compels us to find the inner path after many wanderings. In an unexpected moment, among the animal impulses, in the 'night', in the darkness of unconsciousness, our self-awareness is born, just as the Holy Child was born in a manger, among animals, in the 'night', in darkness. And man sets out on the great path, he decides to journey from the first awakening of consciousness in the Self to the paradisiacal universal consciousness, to the goal. And as he gradually grows conscious in himself on this long path, so there unfolds within him the ability to control creative energy in all its manifestations and to use it in accordance with his will. If he once reaches the highest level, the source of divine power, he will be able to transform the lower forms of energy of divine creative power into their higher forms and with the higher spiritual forms of energy he will be able to control and guide the lower forms and to manifest all of these energies through the corresponding nerve centres. Let us come to know this divine power, let us try by its help to climb higher on Jacob's ladder, and by so doing, help sexual energy to transform itself into its higher vibrations, into spiritual power. Where there is consciousness, creative power is at work.

# Chapter 5
# Jacob's Ladder

Those who set out on the path of Yoga with the intention of *renouncing* sexual energy and suddenly want to lead an abstemious life betray that they are not only ignorant of the divine origin of this energy but even of the energy itself! And how is a man to gain control over something, to renounce it with neither sacrifice nor denial if he has not first thoroughly acquainted himself with it and come to terms with it?

As long as one suspects yet untasted potential pleasures in sexuality one cannot and should not renounce one's sex life. One would then live in the belief of having missed or lost something; and however erroneous it may be, this misconception will again and again lure one into sexual experiences. He alone can reach God who has become thoroughly familiar with sexuality and tasted it and all its potentialities to the full, either in this life or in a previous one. Otherwise, if he is ignorant of sexuality, God too will be beyond his reach. Sexual energy is the bearer of life, therefore also a manifestation of God, albeit in the form of matter and at the lowest level! If our aim is to reach God we must start our ascent of Jacob's ladder from the lowest rung (Gen. 28:12). None of the steps can be omitted, and how could one give something up and go on to climb the next step before becoming thoroughly familiar with the previous one?

If I want to extirpate my sexual energy without first having come to know it, then it will turn against me *with all my own power* because *I am* this energy *myself*, even if only unconsciously! For this very reason *its strength is exactly equal to my own*! On no account can I destroy it, for that would mean destroying *myself*. We cannot destroy sexual energy, we can only transform it! We can only *be* it!

55

I must go through the experiences, I must become so thoroughly familiar with sexual energy, with all its vexations and pitfalls that no aspect of this form of creative energy remains hidden to me. It may be that a person has already acquired this experience and was born with it into this life. He does not need to acquire it again. But he must feel this certainty in himself. We can observe that those even at a higher level of spiritual development start their human life as a sexual object, at a lower level in puberty. But then they take only a very short time to pass from adolescence to adulthood, whereas primal man requires perhaps millions of years for the same development. The unicellular organisms take millions of years to ascend through the stages of reptiles, birds and mammalia to man as we know him, while the human embryo passes through all these phases of development from conception to birth in the compressed period of nine months. Thus a man who has attained a higher level can accomplish all the stages of development of sexual manifestation during the brief phase of youth, from the adolescent's most primitive urge to discharge his pent-up sexuality to the superior adult's highest spiritual sense of belongingness founded on love. Naturally there are many exceptions owing to the countless variations of development and differences of levels attained.

If therefore a person has gone through his experiences of sexual energy, either in the past or present life, he will release himself from its bondage, exercise control over it and use it as *creative power*. If, on the other hand, a man who does not know sexual energy and is unable to transform it preserves it by living an abstemious life, then this primal energy will be thrust down into the unconscious and suppressed so that it manifests itself in a perverted way. With incredible cunning it causes people often the most serious *physical and mental* disorders, illnesses and troubles. It is not usually realized that these are due to repressed and curbed sexual energies. It is particularly dangerous when a married couple, or sometimes even only one partner, suddenly decides to lead an abstemious life. Indeed, it is suspicious that this should even be desired. It is advisable to ask oneself first *very honestly* why one suddenly feels like leading a continent life. It often emerges that the real reason is not so much a strong desire for God, as rather the unfulfilled yearning for love and understanding, a general incapacity for life and, stemming from this, also frustrated sexual desires or unpleasant disappointments. Many people are not sufficiently honest with themselves, they have no wish to accept the true reason, they repress it into the unconscious and say that in order to reach God they want to renounce 'everything'. How do these people conceive of 'God' that they want to renounce 'everything' for him? Does this then mean that sexuality is for them 'everything'? So it seems, for this is usually *all* it amounts to. If they really want to renounce 'everything' then let them, to be consistent, live in a cave. But again they do not want this, only in their imagination. Or perhaps in a centrally-heated cave with bathroom?

Let us therefore beware! As long as anyone sees continence as 'total renouncement', as 'total sacrifice', this is the very reason why he should *not* renounce 'everything', why he should *not* wish to give up everything but should first get to know what 'everything' is. With his married partner he should try to experience a sublime devotion based on love and live a healthy, fulfilling, clean sex life. In so doing he must on no account suggest to himself that a healthy sex life is something degrading or defiling! If he does, his attitude is obviously pathological. Nor on the other hand must a continent life be motivated by unconscious revenge on one's partner or on oneself! Revenge due to disappointment, frustration or failure.

*If one has a healthy attitude towards sex life it is in itself never degrading or defiling.* The Bible tells us not to set up bounds and then feel ourselves to be sinners when we transgress them. It is not sexuality that degrades and defiles man, but man who makes of himself an animal and instead of leading a healthy sex life based on true love and togetherness, deliberately distorts it to a brutish, depraved, even perverse end in itself. He defiles himself and degrades both himself and sexuality.

Whoever has set out on the path of Yoga and wants to progress along the inner path, will not distort sexuality to a brutish end in itself. In marriage, in physical union he will not seek the gratification of animal desires, but rather the *manifestation of a higher, spiritual union.* Giving himself physically will neither degrade nor defile him for his act is motivated by a deeper, spiritual desire for oneness, for love. Why then is he expected to begin Yoga with continence at the very outset? If he is not yet able to transform sexual energy, then a forced abstemious way of life can result in extreme nervousness, disharmony, quarrelsomeness, indeed even

57

in a broken marriage, *because sexual energy has not yet been able to find the way to the higher nerve centres.* Married people should bear in mind that it is not *chance* which has led them to marriage, to their particular marriage. They have been brought to this union by their karma and so *it is this very marriage* which quickens their progress. Their karma will indicate when they are mature enough and the time has come to lead an abstemious life and to proceed, hand in hand, in supreme love and mutual understanding. In this way marriage will not be an unbearable burden but will mean mutual assistance and happiness. Should, however, marriage become a heavy burden, an enslavement and an obstacle to progress, then when the karmic time has elapsed and the karmic debt is paid, it will fall from man, like a used garment. Running away from an oppressive situation is never a solution. The problems have to be solved *or else they keep by our side*! Once we have obtained an inner release from such painful unions, there is a transformation in the outer world too and quite unexpectedly the door to freedom is opened. A marriage is not in itself an obstacle on the path of Yoga. Many great saints in the West as well as in India who were married achieved the highest aim. One of the greatest masters in India, Rama Krishna, lived with his wife Sarada Devi till he died, and both became very great yogis. Equally one might list countless holy men and women in the West who, although married, attained the highest degree of holiness, divine all-consciousness, as for instance St Monica, the mother of St Augustine, and many other saints as well as initiated Rosicrucians.

Man sheds physical desire when he reaches maturity. He has got to know the witchery of sexuality and now he sees through it. This power in its lowest form, as sexual energy, continues to interest him only as a link, as a catalyser between spirit and body, as an auxiliary drive towards progress. But he ceases to maintain that he would have to renounce 'everything' in order to reach God. There is no need for man to '*renounce*' or '*forego*' anything! As soon as he is able to transform sexual energy into its higher form, *he preserves it,* and in a higher and much more valuable form. *He loses nothing but gains all.* For the happiness which man experiences, or rather hopes to experience, in sexuality *remains with him once and for all at a much higher level.* Since he does not expend his energy but preserves it, it continues to dwell in him! We do not lose it, we no longer experience it as very transient, short-lived sexual pleasure, but now exclusively in the higher form of a mental and spiritual beatitude, which is ours for ever and cannot be lost because: I AM IT. *Tat tvam asi! That is you!* in the words of the Vedanta philosophy. We cease to experience creative power in the body as sexual energy, as sexual desire and drive, which is no sooner gratified than it vanishes. Now we experience it directly as creative power itself, as creative joy at an ever higher level of consciousness, as an ever mounting, enduring, eternal *state of being.* I no longer *possess* happiness, I am no longer *happy, I am happiness itself!* How can happiness cease to feel happy if it is *itself* happiness? It is entirely a question of consciousness: if I have not yet grown conscious in the *logos,* in life itself, I experience being as sexual energy, as *sexual drive* which is at work in my *body* and is life-giving for a third person. If I am at a higher level of consciousness, I experience *logos,* life, within me as *love,* manifested in my *soul* as a higher emotion. If I have grown conscious in the *logos,* in life itself, I experience it in the *spirit,* in my Self, as a state of self-awareness, as *myself*: I AM IT!

If, however, I have become *logos* itself, life, I have at the same time received an indescribable feeling of deep contentment, which never fades, which never can fade! We have found what we have been seeking with infinite longing since the first awakening, the first dawning of consciousness. We experience the perfect fulfilment, release and resurrection! *I am* unshakeable self-reliance and translucent self-awareness: I know no fear, dread or uncertainty!

According to the level of consciousness attained, the outward form, the name, the experience, the inner state, change. But the essence of this power remains what in reality it always was, divine-creative power, *logos,* which is our own life, our individual Self; it is that within me, which, when I have grown conscious I experience as myself, as I AM. How can death have power over me if *I am life itself? How could life die?*

When we are able to mobilize from their latent, dormant condition the nerve and brain centres which bear the higher vibrations as resistance – for the higher the state of consciousness, the higher the frequencies and vibrations active in the body – then we are also able to direct creative power higher or lower on Jacob's ladder as we please and to use it at our discretion. The higher the manifestation, the higher the frequencies and tension and the greater

59

the beatitude. The high tension lifts our consciousness in ever-mounting states, nearer and nearer to God. We can only experience God as '*I am that I am*'; as Moses the great initiate who spoke face to face with God said, the name of God is: 'I AM THAT I AM. . . .' Unfortunately people fail to understand what he meant by that.

Let us bear in mind that our models, in the West the great saints and in the East the great masters, the *rishis*, would never have been so foolish as to discard, sacrifice and renounce sexual pleasures if they had been *real and lasting* pleasures. They attained the goal, divine consciousness, and with it a thousandfold higher happiness and supernal fulfilment! The question is simply whether we are seeking a very transient or an eternally lasting happiness. For the pleasures of sex are inevitably subject to time. We know beforehand that we shall in any event lose this happiness and these pleasures sooner or later, whether we like it or not. The greater the happiness, the greater the loss when the time has run out. If, on the other hand, I do not expend this energy through the body, but *become conscious in it*, since I myself am it, if I can attain the state whereby I can again *be* sexual energy, then I shall no longer lose this happiness, for I am it! And the 'Self' is eternal and does not fade with the decay of the body. *It has merely projected and manifested itself in the body as sexual energy and withdrawn again.* But if in my consciousness I become identical not with the projection, the manifestation, but with that which projects, with the manifester, which is my own true being, then I consciously bear life within me. I am it! And the Self is eternal. Thus the joys of the Self are also eternal!

A person who cannot experience life, *logos*, with his conscious mind because these maximum frequencies would still be too much for his nerves, that is to say, someone who is in the transitional period of gradual development, should certainly lead a healthy sex life based on spiritual oneness. Through sexual union two people can afford each other much love and happiness, even if it is a very transient happiness. It in no way degrades them and indeed helps them to build up an intimate relationship and to share in true and sublime experience. And Nature exploits their yearning for love and fulfilment, bewitches them with her spell and promises them the highest happiness through sexuality in order to create further generations. If two people have sought sexual union out of true love and an inner spiritual affinity, and tasted it to the full, then togetherness and love still remain as consolation after sexual fulfilment. For how long? That is another question. For whenever they yielded to the sexual desires, giving them full rein, they found that in the very moment of physical gratification, when they thought that 'now' the promised happiness was coming, it suddenly slipped from them and was gone. And what is more, they expended their own energies for this self-deception. In most cases people seek a sexual relationship not because of a desire for inner union, but for sensual pleasure and physical enjoyment. Afterwards they are left with nothing but a vast emptiness and a feeling of boredom, as we can observe with many couples, young and old. But Nature requires progeny for the propagation of life, and man in his loneliness and forlornness seeks understanding and love in sexuality. Again and again he falls into Nature's trap as long as he does not realize that that is not what he was really seeking, and that sexuality cannot give him what he longs for. Only then, perhaps hand in hand with his life-partner, will he turn ever more attentively to the spiritual path.

Enlightened men have become aware of all this. They have seen through the sham pleasures of sexuality and know that man can constantly bear the ultimate joy, ecstasy and beatitude as a *lasting state* of self-awareness, that he himself can *be* this, provided he does not expend sexual energy but uses it to stimulate, wake and activate the nerve and brain centres still resting in a latent condition. It enables man in his true being to become conscious in God, to attain divine all-consciousness. As the drops of water that are in the sea, that *are* the sea, so man may rest in God, be conscious in God, be God himself. Did not Christ say: 'Is it not written in your law, I said, Ye are gods?' (St John 10:34 and Psalm 82:6.)

# Chapter 6

# The Judas Betrayal

As we have stated in the previous chapter, an abstemious life only makes sense if it does us no harm and we can profit from it. Only the person whose valve to the higher nerve centres is open, thus enabling sexual energy to rise up into the higher centres, is capable of a healthy and happy abstemious life without the ill-consequences of repression and can enjoy the exceptional rewards and inestimable values of this way of life. Repression is precisely what he avoids, he rather uses his power in a higher, spiritual form which yields incomparably greater happiness than if he were to expend it physically as sexual energy.

A person of such high spiritual standing can also manifest physical love of a very ardent nature. He – and he alone – is able to give free rein to the higher frequencies, not only through the already activated spiritual centres as high spiritual frequencies, but also passionately, by way of the body, through the lower centres in a high tension as sexual energy. He can, however, also expend them through the lower centres in a state of high tension with the physical passion of sexual energy. The sexual tension of a rooster is not to be compared with the high tension of a thoroughbred stallion!

But only the highly developed person runs the risk of lapsing into a dissolute life. The danger inherent in acquired knowledge and capacity is that the conscious abilities can be used in two ways – rightly or wrongly. The person who possesses knowledge wholly or in part is liable to error. Instead of converting sexual energy into its higher form, spiritual-creative power, he can use it like black magic, that is to say, he transforms the spiritual powers into sexual energy, he directs them downwards and identifies them with the body. For this reason it is important that the *higher centres are stimulated and activated in stages*, for only then is there a development of a person's moral power that is parallel to, or let us say, in balance with, his creative-spiritual powers, thereby protecting him from all aberrations. Certain paths of Yoga involve this danger. Among them, for example, the so-called Kundalini and Tantra Yoga. In these forms the higher nerve and brain centres are wakened by drastic methods, ignoring the possibility of a gradual organic, spiritual, mental and physical development, which is somewhat slower but all the safer for that. That is why a genuine guru – an initiated spiritual teacher – is always very cautious with his disciples. Only a charlatan meddles unscrupulously with these higher, irresistible, all-pervading creative-magical powers.

We call a person a 'white magician', a 'God-man', if, by a steady development along the path of Yoga, he has become conscious at the highest divine level, and, having reached the highest rung on Jacob's ladder, is master of the entire scale of revealed creative power but only in a lawful, divine-moral way and therefore completely impersonally and selflessly, as the instrument of God. He also transmits his high powers into the body, since he lives in a body, but his consciousness does not leave the source, God. His consciousness is one with God and never identifies itself with the body. He consciously remains what he is in reality, in his true being, life, *logos*, God himself.

The black magician on the other hand, who is at a level of consciousness artificially upgraded by the use of magic, but still completely self-centred and morally underdeveloped, acts in just the opposite way to the white magician: he uses the divine powers to satisfy his personal-egoistic ends and his lust. He identifies his consciousness not with God but with the body, and directs the divine powers downwards from the spiritual to the sexual-physical centres. As soon as the spiritual-creative power, which should likewise be put to spiritual-creative use through the activated higher nerve and brain centres, is directed downwards and abused for personal, physical-egoistic ends, one acts as a black magician.

The fundamental difference between a 'white' and a 'black' magician is that a black magician has command over the divine powers, while the white magician puts himself at their command;

they use him as an instrument. The white magician has become completely impersonal and thus can no longer act as a person. His person no longer exists! Rather, since his consciousness is identical with God, the divine will acts in him and through him. The black magician with his personal-egoistic way of life devotes himself to the passions and pleasures of the body. In so doing he squanders, betrays and kills divine power, *logos*, his divine SELF. He too could work miracles with his high powers, but by betraying them, his own true Self – God – he finally destroys and kills himself. Black magicians always suffer a dreadful death! The Bible describes this betrayal in the story of Judas.

In order to understand the Judas story correctly, we must first know that the Bible is full of allusions to the cosmic implications, therefore to astrological truths. Already in the Old Testament we find references to astrology, as for instance in Ezekiel's vision in one of the most important passages of the Bible. Ezekiel beholds the universe as a vast, square linen cloth spread out, and he sees the four 'animals' at its four corners: the lion, the bull, the cherub and the eagle. These are the four corners of the universe, the four most important signs of the zodiac: Leo, Taurus, Aquarius and eagle.[1] In its lower form the latter is termed Scorpio. We find the same four signs of the zodiac in the symbolic representation of the four Evangelists: St Mark – Leo, St Luke – Taurus, St Matthew – Aquarius and St John – eagle, in its lower form Judas–Scorpio. In his First Epistle to the Corinthians (15:41), Paul too speaks of the effects produced by the radiation of the celestial bodies: 'There is one glory of the sun, another glory of the moon, and another glory of the stars: for one star differeth from another star in glory.'

The rays, the frequencies of the zodiac sign Scorpio, correspond to the frequencies of creative power, which is represented in its higher octave, in its spiritual form, as a soaring eagle by John the Apostle, *who has his head on Christ's breast*. In its lowest form as sexual energy, as the self-destructive scorpion, it is symbolized by Judas. Christ – *logos* – prophesies of Judas: 'He that eateth bread with me hath lifted up his heel against me.' And: 'One of you shall betray me. . . . He it is, to whom *I* shall *give* a sop, when I have *dipped* it.' Sexual energy, the bearer of life, Judas, who 'hath a

[1] cf. Elisabeth Haich, *Initiation*, Allen and Unwin.

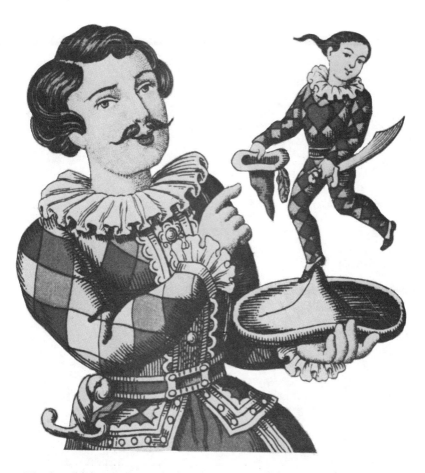

The last, highest tarot card, the great Self, which is sexless because it unites the two poles in its consciousness, makes the homunculus, which is a physical being and belongs to a sex, dance on its hand like a little marionette, as an agent of manifestation, in accordance with his role in the earthly-material world.

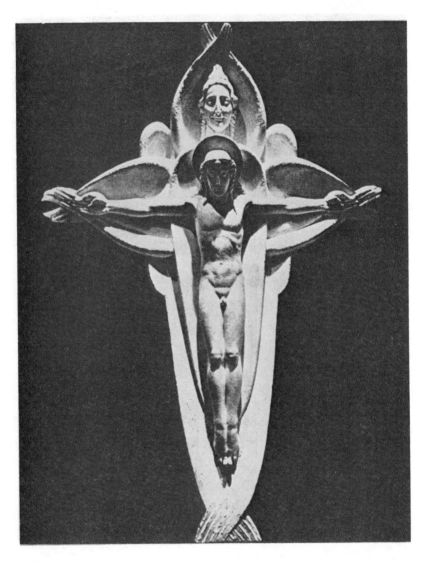

Mestrovic: the eternally crucified Christ: Ottavice. The unconscious man does not know that GOD, who is in reality his true, higher Self, dwells in his unconscious.

purse', is nourished by the creative principle, Christ, 'and when he had dipped the sop, he gave it to Judas Iscariot', and Judas betrays him with a *kiss*: 'Jesus said unto him, Judas betrayest thou the Son of man with a kiss?' 'Kiss' is an erotic act, that is, sexuality. The man of black magic who is already in possession of his creative powers – of the 'purse' – and nevertheless identifies himself with the body, that is to say, directs his spiritual powers downwards, expends the spiritual powers converted into sexual energy in physical pleasure, as end in itself, expends his Christ – his creative-magical *logos* powers – he betrays him, he surrenders, him to the level of matter. Judas sold Christ for thirty pieces of silver – these are the thirty degrees of the zodiac sign Scorpio, which has the same vibration as the sexual organs and for this reason symbolizes the sexual organs and sexual energy. At the moment when the divine, betrayed and expended by Judas, dies on the Cross (the Cross symbolizes the world of matter), Judas must of course also die, but by suicide. As is written in the Bible: at the moment of Christ's death on the Cross, Judas hangs himself and dies also. In killing creativeness he killed himself too, for both the divine-creative energy and sexual energy are *logos* itself, and hence identical with one another. If a man betrays his creative power by dissolute living, by sexual excess and abuse as a means of pleasure, sexuality dies also. He loses his potency, loses his central, suggestive power, he becomes a weak character incapable of resistance; he is shattered, destroyed by the manifold influences of the external world and becomes a prey to his greatest enemy, fear.

Judas killed himself and the creative principle – Christ – and goes on killing it today in every person who abuses his higher qualities and uses his reason to direct his thoughts continuously into the sexual organs; in every person who rouses his senses and sex glands with stimulating foods and drinks, and also with mental aids, pornographic literature, films and plays and who expends his sexual energies in excesses and abuse. And, of course, alcoholism and other addictions go hand in hand with such habits. Experience shows that people who live like this, and also those who squander their creative powers with excessive masturbation, sooner or later – unfortunately rather sooner than later – decline into irresoluteness, spiritual annihilation, darkness and fear. (The occasional masturbation of adolescence does not necessarily have this detrimental consequence. We are talking here only of *perversely excessive* masturbation.)

The simple person with an average level of consciousness is not, and cannot be, a Judas. The possibility of a transformation of energy does not even occur to him. He can direct his energies neither upwards nor downwards, nor can he transform them. If such a person yields to his sexual desires and leads a normal, healthy sex life, he does not sin against the creative principle dwelling in his unconscious, for the simple reason that a *healthy sex life is not a sin*! He does not draw any divine powers down into the body, he does not identify his higher Self, of which he is not yet conscious, with the body and consequently he cannot approach his higher Self, far less abuse it. *Therefore he simply expends physical-sexual powers in a normal way, and not creative-spiritual ones.*

Man's nerve and brain centres are constituted in such a way that they gradually manifest the *logos* energies in a steady development at each stage in the growth of consciousness. Earthly life, however, does not always allow these centres to awake and become active in a regular progression from the lowest to the highest, but in certain cases (unfortunately nowadays in very many cases as a result of civilization), it causes some of the higher centres to emerge from their latent state and become active before the lower centres which should be activated first. This irregularity causes all kinds of mental and physical abnormalities, which can, and alas do, lead to serious disintegration of the ego! The effects of two world wars, the various technical discoveries which man is not nearly mature enough to use, and the great gulf between man and Nature result in our day, as always when great civilizations fall in decay, in the latent nerve centres of an alarming number of people becoming activated out of their proper order, a process which threatens to grow worse and affect not only the white race but also the Asian and African peoples. This is plain to see. Sick-minded people suffering from inferiority complexes and megalomania, who have never developed beyond adolescence, who are still at a very low level of consciousness, but who nevertheless already *possess hypnotic magical powers of a high order*, occupy positions in which they rouse the masses with their activated, electrifying, high-frequency energy and do untold harm to their own and other nations' political and economic life, till *another* person, equally primitive and warped in development, yet possessing magically pervasive energies, ousts them from their position and inflicts, if possible, still greater harm on the community. No wonder that throughout the world conditions of absolute chaos prevail, that people run amok for no apparent reason, and virtually preclude the natural and happy life for which God has given us ample opportunity on earth. Fear, unrest, impotence and misery prevail throughout the world today. Through the Judas traitors who place the supreme spiritual creative powers in the service of their lowest impulses, man has almost completely lost himself.

These are the dangers of the Tree of Knowledge of good and evil! A person who has acquired knowledge without a parallel development of his moral power, who has not yet expanded the sphere of his Self to embrace the community, and has thus not yet converted his egoism into universal love, runs an inherent risk of using his higher powers inversely, directed downwards, unnaturally – as a black magician – and to the great harm of humanity. Only 'knowing' people who *have not preserved the balance* in developing their nerve and brain centres could place the higher spiritual manifestations of the *Self*, such as literature, theatre, film, art, music, in the service of the lowest powers, in the service of unscrupulous demagogy, or sensuality, eroticism, lust, obscene sexuality and pornography. Animals cannot sin through sexuality. When they are roused by the healthy power of Nature they expend it perfectly naturally, breed offspring and also enjoy the pleasures of healthy sexuality. For them that is all there is to it. Man, however, on the one hand still underdeveloped, on the other, already half-aware, uses his reason to think out all kinds of methods of rousing his sensory organs, *even against their will*, and of titillating them merely for the sake of enjoyment and perverse lust. The healthy organs thus grow weak and degenerate, for they have to keep on supplying pleasures beyond their healthy powers. Naturally, the denizens of the underworld exploit human weaknesses for the most sordid kinds of business such as drug dens and other low underworld establishments. Those who, for reasons of unhappiness or addiction to pleasure (which is also rooted in unhappiness), direct their vital energy into their sexual organs which demand ever renewed gratification as a result of constant titillation, have less and less energy for the functions of the higher organs which serve spirituality. The result of this is weakened will-power, constant feelings of apprehension, mental and physical weakness, lowered resistance, inactivity and an incapacity for life. Thus man forfeits his higher spiritual abilities, lapses into senility, and is snuffed out.

# Chapter 7

# The Magical Powers of Suggestion, Hypnosis and Mediumship

In this book frequent use has been and will be made of expressions such as 'magical', 'suggestive-magical' or 'hypnotic-magical' abilities and powers. These and similar expressions require closer definition, for they have been and continue to be used by a number of people with such a variety of meanings that their contours have become indistinct and vague. It is therefore necessary to say something about the meaning of these words in order to avoid misunderstanding.

What is meant by suggestive or hypnotic powers, we have all been able to experience and observe. We know there are people who can impose their will on others – even on animals. We know that this transmission can be effected through methods ranging from simple influence by persuasion, through suggestion, to deliberate hypnosis, by which the 'other' person is subjected to the extraneous will. He becomes an unconscious tool in the hands of the hypnotist, and, completely at his mercy, carries out his will like a marionette devoid of ego and spirit.

Whoever can transmit his will to others is a magical-suggestive or magical-hypnotic person. On the other hand, whoever carries out the will of this 'magician', of the hypnotist, is the medium.

If we observe such transmissions of will merely from the outside, we can perceive only the outward effects. And even if we observe these very closely, we can ascertain nothing save that such phenomena really exist. What renders them possible, and what the powers of the suggestionist, the hypnotist and the medium are in reality can be learned and known only by someone who has experienced and observed these transmissions for himself, *in full awareness*, either as the magical-hypnotic transmitter – that is, as the hypnotist – or as the recipient – as the medium. We lay emphasis on the *conscious* experience, for most people who possess and work with these powers may have become world-famous hypnotists or mediums, but nevertheless had, and have, no inkling of the nature of their own powers. They can describe the phenomena and the laws of these powers which take possession of others merely from the outside, because they have and use these powers not consciously, but unconsciously. They see and observe the effects, but they are ignorant of the power itself and its functions.

It is not in itself easy to gain conscious knowledge of these powers and to observe them. To do so, an innate ability is essential. It is still less easy, once we have attained a fully conscious experience of these phenomena, to explain them in words to those who can have no share in such direct experience. It is as difficult as explaining to a blind man that, although the intellect comprehends certain vibrations as 'vibrations', it cannot *perceive* them as such but that they can be 'seen' quite simply and directly with the eyes. It would be still more difficult to explain that it is not the 'vibrations' one sees – 'vibrations' are invisible – but that we see 'light' without being aware that it is actually made up of measurable vibrations.

The same is true of every mental experience. Only through our individual, direct experiences and states of being can we perceive it and make it conscious within us. The intellect can only understand something; it can never perceive, see, hear, taste or feel and thus experience directly. Yet only by its assistance is it possible to pass on the inner mental experiences, for the intellect alone is able to create and comprehend words and to give insight into what is not direct experience. Only the intellect is able to bridge the gap between ignorance and knowledge. On the basis of direct experience, then, a rational explanation will be attempted of what is meant by suggestion, hypnotism and mediumship.

We know that man receives various rays from the universe and his environment. In the same way he himself emits various energies, being an independent centre, an 'EGO'. He has seven main energy centres – the *chakras* – through which he receives the energies emitted from the cosmos, transforms them and transmits them in seven forms of energy to his body, his surroundings and the outer world. Since these energy centres are generally not yet in an activated but still in a more or less latent condition in men, their function varies according to a man's particular level of development. It therefore stands to reason that the quality and quantity of the total radiation of different people also varies widely. This depends on a man's individual level of development.

We know from scientific wave theory that the waves of the various radiations may reinforce, weaken or even neutralize one another, depending on the relationship between the type and length of the waves. If different waves are superimposed so that their frequencies coincide, they have a mutually strengthening effect; if their frequencies are opposed, however, the effect is weakening or neutralizing because a gap occurs in the continuity. These points of neutralization are scientifically termed 'interference'.

The individual radiations of men naturally work on the same principles, for everything is analogous. Hermes Trismegistus said: 'As above, so below.' They have an effect on their environment and outer world, no matter whether plants, animals or humans are present there. It is a fact that in the presence of loving people everything is animated; plants are fresher and thrive with greater profusion, children and animals reared by such people grow healthy and strong, and all adults near them become healthier, livelier, stronger, indeed happier. On the other hand, there are others in whose presence all plants wither and die and children and animals grow weak and ailing. Avoided by their fellow-men, these people become increasingly lonely and isolated.

Born doctors, nurses, masseurs, gardeners, as well as people in other walks of life, clearly illustrate this beneficial effect. It may be the father of a family, or a mother, a nanny who has grown old with the family, sometimes an 'uncle', a friend or a professional colleague, who is everyone's favourite because he or she has a strikingly animating, beneficial radiation. Such people attract all living creatures and are everywhere the cherished life and soul of their spheres.

What is the secret of these people?

It is this: the higher the frequencies and the shorter the waves which a person emits, the closer they approach certain frequencies, vibrations and rays which cannot be detected scientifically, although we experience them directly and simply call them 'love'. The frequencies of *love* represent the very shortest waves, the very highest frequencies; they are so penetrating that they pierce through, permeate and even transform all other forms of energy.

Nothing and no one can resist these frequencies, nothing can isolate itself from them. They are the highest, divine frequencies, for love is God! People also emit lower frequencies, for each state, feeling, thought, spoken word and deed has a lower or higher radiation and effect. Accordingly, the effect of these manifestations is to attract or repel, strengthen, weaken or destroy, to give or take.

There are people who can perceive these radiations as distinctly and directly as all living creatures see rays of light with their eyes. We can only explain this rationally, by analogies and similes, as telepathy, for instance, can be explained by analogy with radio or television.

A person, like every living creature, therefore emits combined energies and is surrounded by them, just as a lamp is surrounded by its own kinds of radiation – light, heat and so forth. This composite radiation differs with each individual, and the more conscious a man has grown in his true Self, the more powerful the effect of his radiation on his environment, on plants, animals and people. Just as a lamp radiates light and the stronger that light, the greater the luminosity round the lamp, so man is surrounded by his own radiation, and the limit of this is the limit of his mental vision and also of his will. Just as the big lamp shines through the small lamp, but the small lamps are unable to penetrate the big ones, so the man of greater self-awareness illumines less conscious men – he sees them – without their being able to illumine and see him. The history of mankind supplies numerous instances where men of genius have illumined their fellow-men with their spiritual eyes and recognized them clearly, but they in their turn have neither seen nor recognized these giants, indeed they have even frequently abused such men, and sent them to the stake or some other form of death.

Thus the great man sees his fellow-men, but they do not see him. Just as the radiation of the greater man penetrates the lesser man, and his frequencies encounter the other's waves, thereby strengthening or perhaps weakening them, so in the same measure will the other man find him likeable, disagreeable or repulsive. This also holds good when people of the same level of development meet and influence each other. It may happen that, in spite of being at the same level of development, the one is more developed in one direction but has fallen behind in another in which his fellow-man has advanced farther. Consequently, the sum total of their development may be equal, yet depending on their composition, they may have a strengthening, weakening, or – as a result of interference – repelling effect on each other. Mathematical laws operate in man's being, as in the whole of creation, for man is also created in accordance with these laws. For this reason we find each other likeable or disagreeable, if not actually repulsive.

If a person of a higher level of development exerts an influence on an inferior human being, it can happen that the frequencies of the stronger man meet those of the weaker one in such a way that they greatly strengthen certain of his frequencies, causing them to dominate in the weaker man. In other words: the qualities already present in him, which may have been unconscious and weak, if not actually latent, suddenly become alive, conscious and strong, through the analogous radiation of the stronger person. We then say that the stronger person has 'influenced him by suggestion'. When such an influence is exerted on a subject, he does not lose his own will-power, he remains himself since his frequencies also remain what they have been, they remain *his own* emanations. Only certain components of his frequencies have been emphasized, intensified and made conscious by the synchronized vibration of the stronger person. Thus his will-power has not been weakened but roused by the other. There can therefore be no question of his being possessed. Possession, that is to say, the state of hypnosis, obtains only when the stronger person penetrates the weaker one with his frequencies, and through the vibrations which can be reduced to a common denominator in both cases, reaches the weaker man's innermost being, possessing him to such an extent that his will-power dwindles and he yields more and more to the extraneous power, to the stronger person's will. This can go so far that the stronger person, the one who has become the hypnotist, possesses the weaker one, the medium, through the common frequencies so completely that he also forcibly changes the remaining frequencies of the medium, which are *not common* to both, and remoulds them, as it were, in his own image. The medium is thereby ultimately forced to receive so many extraneous frequencies that his own consciousness is suppressed and reduced to a latent condition. There are various stages of this state ranging from simple suggestion by verbal persuasion to total hypnosis and total possession.

Suggestion is therefore a state in which the subject still retains his right of self-determination and accepts the will of the suggestionist in full consciousness.

Suggestion becomes mild hypnosis if the effect of the suggestionist is gradually to weaken and suppress the subject's will until he unconsciously surrenders his right of self-determination, blindly adopts the will of the suggestionist, who has now assumed the full role of hypnotist, and becomes his passive instrument.

In total hypnosis the extraneous vibrations of the hypnotist, forcibly imposed on the medium, have penetrated him thoroughly and taken possession of him, thereby yielding him up in an unconscious state to the hypnotist. In his power the medium becomes a pliable tool, for his consciousness has been forced down to the deepest levels of his unconscious and he automatically executes the hypnotist's will. It is a well-known fact that while this condition of the medium can be used beneficially, say for healing, it can also be used for evil ends.

At this point a very important question arises. We have seen that the stronger person, namely the *more conscious one* (for a person's strength always depends on the extent to which he has grown conscious), can instil his will into the weaker person by suggestion, indeed he can even subjugate him completely to his will, that is to say, he can hypnotize him. But how does it happen that a very conscious, and therefore a very powerful, individual may exercise little or no influence over his fellow-men, while there are plenty of people who, although neither very conscious nor highly developed, nevertheless have a strong, suggestive and hypnotic influence over others? There are plenty of examples of great geniuses, both past and present, who have exercised no suggestive power whatsoever, still less any hypnotic power, over their fellow-men, while on the other hand, average men of moderate abilities have frequently acquired and exploited hypnotic power over vast numbers of people, or they have become famous hypnotists effecting countless cures by means of their hypnotic gift. Again others have influenced weak characters in a criminal way.

The answer to this question is provided by mathematics.

We do not intend to discuss here in detail the theory of numbers or magic of numbers. Yet if we wish to understand better the inner laws of the human being, the simplest way is to make use of numbers, since man – like the whole of creation – is created in accordance with mathematical laws.

We know that in the series of natural numbers, infinitely many are divisible not only by the number *one* and by *themselves* but also by other numbers. But we know too that there are infinitely many numbers – even large ones exceeding millions – which are divisible only by the number *one* and by *themselves* and no other number, that is, they are indivisible. In the theory of numbers these are known as 'prime numbers'.

As mentioned before, men, just like any energy centre, emit different vibrations and frequencies. These have a definite frequency which characterizes the person. Since men manifest endless variations of character, their frequencies are likewise so innumerable and varied that they can just as easily belong to the category of the factorable – divisible – numbers as to that of the non-factorable – indivisible – prime numbers. If we remember the law that the waves of various frequencies can only influence one another if they share certain affinities, similarities or even identities, we shall understand that *a stronger person can only exert influence upon another – a weaker person – if the frequency of the stronger person is divisible by that of the weaker one.*

Now we can understand that a person at a lower level of development than another may have a much greater measure of suggestive power than other men – he may even have hypnotic power – *because his frequency belongs to the numbers divisible by many others.* Let us take, for example, the number sixty. It is not a big number in the infinite series of numbers and yet it can be divided by *twelve* numbers – by *one, two, three, four, five, six, ten, twelve, fifteen, twenty, thirty,* and by *itself.* Thus, a person whom we could characterize with the number *sixty* can have a suggestive or hypnotic influence on *twelve* different types of people. If, however, we take as our example the number 257, we find that although more than four times sixty, this number contains only the number *one* and *itself* without a remainder, but no other number by which it could be divided. It is therefore an indivisible prime number. A person characterized by this, or another even greater prime number, cannot exert suggestive or hypnotic power over anyone, at however high a level he may be. He remains isolated and powerless among his fellow-men, because his energies do not correspond with others and are therefore blocked. There are plenty of other examples where, in contrast to a highly developed person, another at a much lower level of development – a simple, primitive man – emits great suggestive and hypnotic power because the highly developed man is characterized by, say, the number 65,537 and the primitive man, for example, by the number 12. Although 65,537 is a relatively high number, it is still an indivisible prime number, and thus has no access to others. On the other hand, the number 12, low though it may be, has access to six numbers, for it is divisible by six different numbers (half of itself!). Hence, this person has suggestive power with regard to six types of people – at a lower level of consciousness than himself, of course. In general, the average person is not at a high level of consciousness. So we can see why it is possible that superior geniuses should frequently stand solitary and alone, without any contact or suggestive power, while undeveloped people of limited intelligence – alas very often a simple fortune-teller – exercise mysterious power. Naturally, a person on a high level whom we could characterize, for instance, with the number 30,240 can exert legitimate power over great multitudes of people, often quite unintentionally. Everywhere he will meet with sympathy and support because very few people are able to escape from his penetrating, suggestive and hypnotic powers. Multitudes of people will vibrate in harmony with him, whether they wish to or not, because the number 30,240 is divisible by *ninety* numbers This person will have access to ninety types of people and will thus command vast hypnotic power. In the same way it is understandable that some people will hate him from the bottom of their hearts! Yet this number is still less than half that of our previous example, 65,537!

If we look at exceptional men such as Moses, Buddha, Confucius and Jesus, we can imagine what high frequencies these 'white magicians' must have had, and with how high a frequency, if we had the means to measure it, we should have to characterize these and all other great teachers and masters! The works of these greatest of men were influential not only in their time and sphere – when and where they lived – but have continued to reverberate in the atmosphere of the whole world, through time and space, down to the present day and in all eternity.

I omit instances of black magicians intentionally.

And now the question arises: what is the difference, with regard to the numbers, between superior highly developed people whom we call 'white magicians', and those who are their mirror image, also superior and highly developed, but who practise black magic, who have always existed and still exist in our time?

Any person who suppresses the right of self-determination of others or even deprives them of it in order to use them as puppets in the service of his selfish ends, is already a black magician. Each man can, and should, fight with human weapons; but not with magical powers and certainly not with the vast magical power acquired by the transformation of sexual energy. A superior person may use these powers only in the interest of the great whole in which – as he must know – all of us, himself included, are only one minute cell. If a person develops steadily, if his latent energy centres are activated in the correct sequence, then, even before he is able to use his highest energy centres, his inner spiritual eyes will already be open to this truth, and he will have no desire whatsoever to use his magical-hypnotic power egoistically, for his personal ends, out of power-mania. Not because he is, or wants to be, 'so selfless', but because he feels completely at one with the great whole and out of *sheer egoism* has regard for its good and *serves* this end with all his magical powers. *For there is only one kind of love: selfish love.* The sole difference is *who* and *what* I incorporate into the sphere of my selfish love. It can include a person, an animal, a family, any social group or association, any nation, the whole earth or the universe. Then people call this same 'selfish love' 'selfless love', because I have extended the circle of my self-love to include the whole universe. But the love has not changed at all, it has only developed. At first I love myself, then finally I love the whole universe like myself, better expressed, *as myself*, because I have developed and in the course of this my love has also developed and I recognize that *I am* the whole universe! – *Tat tvam asi!*

The 'white magician' will therefore never wish to suppress another man's consciousness, to assert his own will over him and to enslave him. Quite the contrary. He will even help to develop the consciousness of other men so that they will then *voluntarily* enlist

77

themselves in the service of divine intentions and plans. The white magician *remains at his own centre, but from there, from within himself, he radiates animating powers of love and thus life itself*. He also allows the other person to *remain* free and uninfluenced *within his centre* so that he not only preserves his right of self-determination, but with the help of the white magician develops to an even higher level.

The black magician on the other hand, out of sheer power-mania, uses his creative energies to lure people under his spell and to use them as slaves. Through suggestion or hypnosis he seizes the other person's centre and makes him serve his personal, selfish ends as a satellite in orbit around him, regardless of whether his victim is mentally or physically destroyed in the process.

The white magician remains within his own centre, radiating from there to the whole outer world the divine-magical power of *love*. The black magician intrudes into the other man's innermost being, eats himself into his soul, penetrates him with his will, destroys him and makes of him an unconscious automaton dancing attendance upon him.

However high the frequencies emitted by the white magician, he remains with his consciousness within the number *one*, within the number of God, which is itself indivisible, but which can divide all numbers *ad infinitum*. He exerts his influence on every living creature through the number *one*, with the most irresistible radiation and power of *love*. As we have said, the white magician remains with his consciousness within the number *one* and radiates from there to infinity. Thus he is completely *impersonal*. The black magician steps out of the *undivided whole* into plurality, he attains the very high number of knowledge and power and identifies himself with the very high number of his own, personal frequencies, thereby becoming a super-individual concerned solely with the promotion of his own, personal interests. That all the evil wrought by a black magician finally rebounds on himself, and that he comes to a dreadful end, stands to reason.

The number *one* is the number of God. Without the number *one* there is no other number. This number is the beginning, just as without God there is no beginning, no creation. The number *one* cannot be divided. All other numbers are divisible by the number *one*, because every number contains it without a remainder and is penetrated by it. Even the highest prime number must submit without resistance to penetration by the number *one*, just as God penetrates the most isolated man with his irresistible power of *love*, infuses him and destroys the isolating crust with his fire.

God is contained without a remainder in the whole of creation, from the smallest to the greatest creature, because God is the father of the whole creation. In the same way the number *one* is the father of all numbers!

The number of God is the number *one*. Yet there is a number which transcends the understanding of the human, finite intellect, which is the reflection of the number *one* in the infinite. Just as the number *one* is the starting-point of the entire creation, so this unimaginable number is the fulfilment, the end of creation. Just as every number can be divided by the divine number one, so this number of fulfilment and the infinite can be divided by every number. No scientist can calculate this number, because it is the number of the infinite and yet it exists as the all-embracing, infinitely great reflection of the number *one*. Just as no number can exist without the number *one*, so by the same token, there can be no number that is not contained without a remainder in this unimaginable number of the infinite.

God is love, and the frequencies of love are so high that they can be expressed only by this number: it contains all other numbers in itself and is therefore the number of the infinite. Just as eternity is beyond the limits of time, yet can be expressed only through time, which belongs to the finite creation, so we can surmise the infinitely great number of God's frequencies – of love – only through knowledge of the limited finite numbers. Eternity itself is not subject to time, yet time is part of eternity. Thus we find the infinitely many finite numbers in the infinite, in eternity, which does not know the finite and fragmentation: in God.

While the number *one* is the number of God and expresses his invariability, indivisibility and eternity, it still forms every number *ad infinitum*. In the same way as God is omnipresent, creating and animating all things without being touched by his creation, so the number *one* forms all numbers, indeed is prerequisite for their existence, without being touched by them and their compounds. And as the number *one*, the creator of all numbers is the starting-point, so its reflection is the number of the infinite and fulfilment,

79

which contains all numbers in itself, the end of all creation and the finite. At this point there remains only *nothingness*, from which the universe has emerged and into which it will be absorbed and disappear. Our EGO is God, the number *one* in us. But in fulfilment this number *one* extends to the number beyond human understanding, the number of the infinite. Man's path leads from the number *one*, from the birth of consciousness to the number of the infinite, where we embrace the whole *universe* in *one consciousness*.

Just as the first primal sound of the creation itself created all remaining sounds by its own harmonic tones, and just as we hear only this single, great primal sound with its all-pervading power when we simultaneously sound its harmonics, so we shall become the number *one*, the one, single, divine *Self* permeating the whole universe by animating all existing frequencies. And it will come to pass that all men, all living creatures, the whole of creation will be penetrated, kindled, animated, wakened and called to a new eternal life in God by the all-penetrating power of the primordial number *one*.

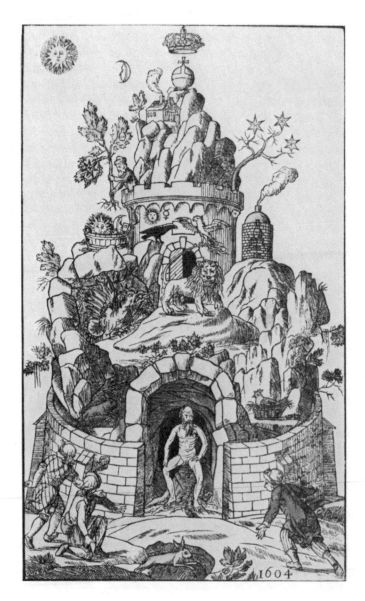

At the top left of this picture the sage creates the philosopher's stone by planting his tree of life in a tub filled with the elixir of life. This is constantly heated by the fire of the dragon – sexual energy – in order to make the sage's tree of life blossom. (Rosicrucian representation.)

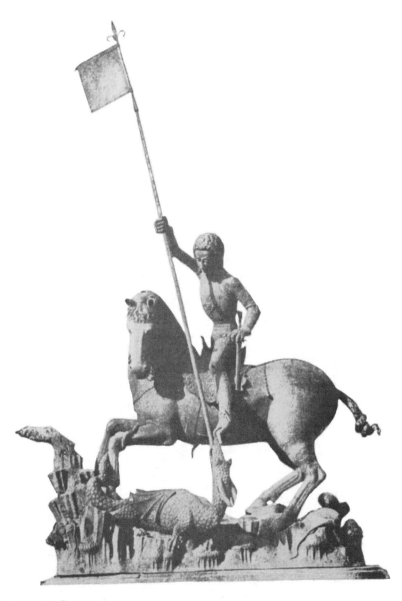

St George has attained all-consciousness and conquers the dragon – sexual energy. But he does not slay him, for he needs the fire, the strength of the dragon, in order to reach GOD. (Brother Kolozsvari, Hradcany Castle, Prague.)

# Chapter 8

# The Seven Rungs of Jacob's Ladder

As long as man is still an unconscious creature, his *logos*-powers operate in him at an unconscious level, automatically and in accordance with the laws of Nature, as in the case of animals. His sexual energy manifests itself within him as a purely animal-physical urge, driving him to rid himself of the unpleasant nervous tension caused by accumulated potency. Accordingly, his state of consciousness is nothing but an animal urge for release. He has no inkling of love, for he is still unable spiritually to experience and manifest his unconscious, dormant desire for it. His higher centres are still in a latent condition, his heart is dead. From this apparent death he is awakened by his sex urge. In a state of physical excitement, stimulated by his sexual energy, he instinctively seeks a partner. Nature deceives him. For sexual excitement serves the sole purpose of procreation, of propagating the vast current of life in order to attain the great goal, the spiritualization of the earth. Primitive man is ignorant of all this. He pursues his sexual desires for gratification. Usually, however, the laws of human civilization and general moral codes prevent gratification immediately the sex drive makes itself felt. Whether he likes it or not, he is compelled to postpone fulfilment for some time. Even among the primitive Negro and bushman tribes, the young men who have just reached maturity must restrain their healthy sexuality till the great ceremony. Only then are they initiated into the secrets of sexuality. Whether in other parts of the world or with the white races of the West, it is a fact that man must first wait with his urge till he eventually finds an opportunity of gratifying his sexual desires, while an animal assailed by sexual desire seeks a suitable partner and usually finds one straight away. Man is required, then, to wait some time. During this waiting period the tension mounts within him and, since it does not find immediate release, this energy tries to discharge itself in another way, through the nerve channels. The unreleased tension builds up and thus man is charged with ever-quickening vibrations and frequencies. If, however, the frequencies of an energy increase, *the energy is also no longer what it was previously.* Thus the first transformation of sexual energy, however small, has already occurred!

The new tension, increased by accumulation, with its higher frequencies now no longer operates solely on his sexual organs, but also on his higher organs which are able to sustain and manifest the increased frequencies. The drive has the added effect of rousing his intellect, he racks his brains for an idea, a solution. Physical desire wakens his consciousness and thus the first glimmer, however faint, in the dawn of awareness has been achieved. Sooner or later he also finds the chance to release his sexual desire, so he is not required to repress it, and yet, at the same time, the first step in the transformation of sexual energy has been taken. Of course, this does not happen as simply and quickly as appears from this description, and although the effect too varies with each individual, the result is the same.

As has been said already, man can develop certain pathologically nervous, often very dangerous inner states, known in modern psychiatry as 'repressions'. This happens when his higher nerve centres have not yet been activated and he is consequently still unable to transform his sexual energies into creative power, yet leads a continent life. But if in the same state of development he restrains his sex drive only for a short period and then gives it free rein, he will not cause repression. In his yet unconscious state he has taken the first steps on the path of transforming sexual energy, quite unintentionally. What compelled him to do so? Unsatisfied sexual energy. We can therefore say that the very sexual energy within us helps to transform – sexual energy. Through the very lack of gratification it has heightened its tension, and by a mental effort has already elevated and expanded the consciousness in some small measure. In this way, whenever a person is unable to fulfil his sexual desires on the first impulse, he climbs the next rung on the ladder of growing consciousness. He ascends step by step till he reaches the stage where he becomes inwardly conscious, not only of his physical desire, but also of his Self. Yet the driving force does not cease to work in him; it urges him on with its ever-recurring, heightened tension, assisting and compelling him to experience by degrees correspondingly higher states of consciousness. Gradually he will reach the level, where, in a state of sexual excitement, he will not feel a purely animal desire to spend himself, but will experience and manifest the first intimation of a human togetherness, even if it is merely in the still primitive form of physical devotion. Even though this may be no more than impassioned possessiveness and subjection, there nevertheless exists a new human relationship between himself and the partner whom he has got to know more closely through sexual intercourse. The first tokens of tenderness, the first symptoms of love appear. Thus his dead heart is in time warmed through and wakened. The purely sexual urge gives way to the desire for fulfilment at a higher level, at the second level of manifestation – that of being in love. And since, moreover, he begins to emerge from the nondescript masses as an individual, he is thus also no longer indiscriminately content with any partner, but seeks one more suited to him and to his developing taste. Several lives may pass during the course of this development from an uncouth, unconscious, primitive man to the attainment of this level. Eternity is long enough. . . .

The primitive man, still trapped in the prison of slow, natural development over eons, may start at the third level of consciousness only in some future life. Then he no longer gratifies his sex urge *indiscriminately*. He becomes more selective and also tries to please his partner. His relationship to the member of the opposite sex changes to a mixture of sexual desire and sense of togetherness coupled with possessiveness, which although primitive and selfish, is already an inferior form of love. His originally purely sexual urge has turned into amorousness, which ties him to a *particular person*.

This amorousness is further fanned by the fire of his sexual energy, which through waiting has intensified. On the other hand, his sexual desire is heightened by the hope of winning this one person of his choice. Such sexual energies, having been raised to a higher level, act with an intensified effect on the higher centres if, in discharging, they encounter obstacles. We could list numerous instances from the history of mankind which prove what ingenious and cunning feats lovers can be made to perform by their frustrated sexual desires if, in spite of all obstacles, they are determined to win the unattainable partner. Frustrated sexual energy has a very stimulating effect on the higher centres, above all on the intellect. The kindled intellect promises the lovers the highest happiness through gratification of their sexual desires. Thus their amorousness is further enhanced, and for reasons of love, if nothing else, they get married. If a man has attained his goal and married, sexual energy finds its outlet free of restraint. Usually, however, sharp-witted heroes and heroines of love then turn into satisfied, boring philistines, till such time as providence compels them to renewed transformation of energy. The husband – caught in Nature's trap – begins to think more about his work in order to ensure a better life for his family, if not entirely because of the pleasure work affords him. He seeks to achieve more. In so doing he is impelled to direct more energy into the higher channels, through which he discharges a greater proportion of these creative energies. Thus the average man is compelled by his sexual energy and his amorousness to direct part of his driving force to the intellectual level and to con-vert it into mental effort. He gradually comes to know the pleasure of creative work, and thus, for the first time, he experiences a kind of self-confidence. His self-awareness grows and expands. Time and habit transform his possessiveness and lust for his life-partner, who by this time has become the mother of his children, into a spiritual-human bond, a loving, domestic harmony, an already higher, more selfless form of love.

Thus unconsciously, and without noticing it, he directs his sexual energies increasingly into higher centres, and gradually attains the next, the fourth level in the development of conscious-ness. He begins to receive and emit ever higher frequencies. These rouse and open still other higher nerve centres; he begins to think even more, and no longer merely about how better to gratify his impulses and how to obtain yet further sensual-sexual pleasures and delights. He also starts taking an interest in higher things. He seeks to give his life more substance, he gradually becomes more individual, he knows that in physical love, too, only an understand-ing partner with whom he shares a spiritual affinity can give him gratification. He looks for, and expects from his lover a similar way of thinking and similar taste. But his increased demands in love narrow the choice of suitable partners, and thus too his chances of full sexual gratification. The more refined his taste, the less easy his gratification. His frustrated and pent-up sexual energies force his consciousness to climb faster, even higher, and also to perceive higher frequencies. In so doing, he activates the next highest nerve centre. His interest turns to knowledge! Thus he reaches the fourth level and grows into it. He begins to study, to learn, he wishes to unravel the mysteries of the world. His mental horizon widens. His creative powers no longer manifest themselves solely through the body as sexual energy, but as emotional and intellectual powers and as strengthened will-power. He 'gets on' in his career, he may hold a leading position, he stands out from the masses. Through carrying a higher vital tension, and becoming conscious at higher frequencies, he also directs higher vibrations into his sexual organs, causing a correspondingly *large increase in his physical-sexual potency! The higher his level of consciousness, the higher and more powerful the energies which man is also able to direct to his lower nerve centres and organs,* and correspondingly greater the pleasures of sexual union! For this, however, he requires a partner as superior as himself. In his love-life he seeks an understanding, exceptional woman who is his equal, and with whom he can form a close spiritual and intellectual relationship. He already has the experience, and knows that *perfect gratification of mind and body and the joy of genuine happiness are only possible with a worthy and equal partner. She must have the ability to follow him into the greatly increased frequencies, and, fired by a passionate yet sublime love, to reciprocate these with her whole being!* He is already aware of the vast difference between quantity and quality and also lives accordingly, because he can no longer live in any other way!

It is extremely sad indeed if a person of a higher level of development is capable of expending and imparting very high tensions in loving and yet his partner is unable to follow him. How dreadfully alone such a person feels!

On the shore at low tide one finds countless mussels lying around, which have been washed up by the waves and dried by the sun. As a child I used to try and piece these halves together to make them one again. There were many simple ones, quite smooth and with a smooth, flat rim. Even if two halves did not belong to the same mussel, they were usually a good match and I could close them. Less common were the mussels which were not flat, but corrugated on the outside and the rim. They were much more beautiful and individualized. I could only put these together properly if the two halves were of the same mussel, only if they belonged together. They did not harmonize with the half of another mussel. . . .

People, too, are like this. The primitive man could find many partners with whom he could share a peaceful life. The husband earns the living, the wife looks after husband and children, together they bear the burdens of life in peace. Habit, their children and the family unite them, but without deep spiritual harmony, for the very reason that they are not yet spiritual, not yet individual. The more spiritual, the more unique and individual a person becomes, the more important it is for him that his marriage-partner matches his level of development in every respect. The more defined a person's character, the less possible it is for him to live together with a lover who does not suit him, and there can be no peace between the two. The higher a man's level, the more essential it is for him that his partner's intellectual level, her intelligence, way of thinking, taste, right down to every detail of their love-making, indeed her whole nature, suit him perfectly. Only with this woman can he also have a pleasurable, gratifying sexual encounter, in which both parties experience perfect oneness in mind, soul and body.

Thus man slowly grows into the fifth level. At this level of consciousness he has reached the point where he can manifest his creative powers in the form of sexual, as well as spiritual, mental and intellectual energies, and beyond that, as ever-increasing iron will-power. He radiates his powers, partly already in a purely intellectual, partly in a spiritual and partly in a physical form, in the direction of his current interest, according to his state of consciousness. He has activated his nerve and brain centres which are capable of bearing higher, purely intellectual energies and high tensions. The resistance of his nerves and body has so increased that he can sustain the high intellectual frequencies without detriment, and also manifest them as sexual energy through his body. He is passionate in his love – it emanates from an inner, spiritual harmony. His sexual organs, powerful and resistant from birth, are also correspondingly capable of manifesting high, passionate tensions. He has become creative; all the valves at five levels, from intellectuality to physical manifestations, are open. Only two further brain centres, which will at some time in the future bear and manifest the very highest, divine frequencies, remain in a latent condition.

If a person radiates all his powers uniformly, then there has automatically also been a uniform development of his organs of mànifestation, and consequently, a supremely intellectual person lives in a beautifully formed, healthy, strong body. This is the level, at which for the first time – *if he so wishes* – man is able to give up his sexual manifestation without resulting harm, pathological nervousness and other difficulties, because he is able to manifest his power at the higher levels free from restraint. Wherever he turns his interest, that is to say, his consciousness, his high creative power manifests itself through corresponding nerve or brain centres and through the suitable organs. He can manifest his sexual energy and experience it as love, he can beget children, or, if he turns his interest to the world of ideas, he can manifest supremely intellectual, creative-suggestive thoughts and scatter them as fertile seeds. He has become intuitive and suggestive, his hypnotic-magical abilities unfold and come into play. We have only to remember those great geniuses who were not only sexually very potent and experienced passionate love, but also penetrated the whole of mankind with their high, creative ideas born of inspiration. They begot *intellectual children* with mankind, they created new worlds and altered the course of history, just as they could give a woman happiness with their physical powers and beget children with her.

We know from history that during creative work great geniuses have often abstained from manifestations of love for many months. They expended all their energies in intellectual manifestation; afterwards, however, they again manifested passionate love and devotion with unchanged potency. These men, at the fifth level in the development of consciousness, already experience creative power as a state of being. They experience it as pleasure in work, as existence, and their influence is magical-creative in every respect. It does not matter whether such a man manifests his energies as a scholar, politician, statesman, ruler, philosopher, or as a performer, composer, painter, sculptor or author. The impact of his influence is the measure of his greatness. It is of no consequence where and when these men lived and worked – or are living and working at the present time. They are above time and space! Their work shines as divine light over the whole earth at all times, and this light diffuses its brightness over the world of finiteness and transience. An Aristotle, a Pythagoras, Plato or Plotinus is as much above time and space as a Spinoza, Leibniz, Kant, Shakespeare, Goethe, Michelangelo, Leonardo da Vinci, Titian, Rembrandt, Rubens or a Beethoven, Mozart, Bach or a Galileo, Edison, Marconi, Paracelsus, Hahnemann and other titans of this world. They looked into creation, brought down to us and revealed what they had experienced at the higher levels. 'There is no greater happiness than to approach the Godhead and bring it down to men,' wrote Beethoven in a letter to the Wegelers. How great his spiritual love that for him the highest happiness was to bring down happiness to men!

Many of these great geniuses experienced physical love and enjoyed it to the full. It is, however, neither necessary nor possible to list here the number of titanic men who have transformed human love into divine love. I recall for instance Plato – it is after him that we term ideal love 'Platonic' – and Dante, who created an image of pure, heavenly love in Beatrice, in his Divine Comedy. We observe too that many of these men were deeply religious – without bigotry – and yearned for God. And we know that many of these giants could abstain from manifesting sexual energy over a long period and remain harmonious and healthy, free from repression. Beethoven was once asked why he did not marry: 'How could I write my music if I were to expend my energies in conjugal life,' was his reply.

Man just cannot serve two masters. He must decide whether to direct his creative powers into the higher or the lower centres. Truly great men have never lived licentiously. On the other hand, incarnations of The Rake never have, nor will, become great men. We find this truth very graphically symbolized in the biblical account of Samson: Samson possessed incomparable and invincible magical power, which radiated from his higher brain centres, thus from his skull, like a thick mane of hair. This power, which also endowed him with his legendary physical strength, vanished like shaved hair when he directed his magical-creative powers into the lowest centres and used them up in sexual intercourse with Delilah. At the same time he was 'blinded', he lost his spiritual vision and spiritual freedom: he was put in 'prison', locked up in himself and isolated. Because he *found the way back to himself* in 'prison', and retained his energies for himself, he was able to transform them once more into creative-magical powers which the reactivated higher centres once again emitted. His strength-giving hair began to grow again, grew long, and he once more became capable of superhuman feats and was able to destroy the royal palace – the identification of consciousness with the realm of matter. In this way he was released from his suffering.

Thus human consciousness gradually raises itself to the sixth step of Jacob's ladder. At this level we find the prophets, the saints, the great teachers of the West and the great masters and *rishis* of the Orient. They have become familiar with creative power at each level and obtained complete mastery over it. They know that to expend this divine power in the body would undeniably be a sad loss to those who use vital energy as creative power and are consequently able to know and experience the joys and happiness of the spirit. Sexual desire has fallen away from them like a ripe fruit from a tree. Their sexual organs are as strong and healthy as those of other men, since it is the spirit that builds the body, and the power of the spirit reveals itself in a perfect body. Since, however, the body obeys the spirit, the sexual organs work for their own body, providing it with the hormones necessary to maintain its health and strength and keep it supplied with ever-renewed energy. In the bodies of these people sexual potency is in a state of dormancy. The energies which would stimulate these organs to procreation are directed into higher nerve and brain centres and expended in a divine-creative way as spiritual energies. These men give up human-creative activity, they neither write literary works nor compose music for the public, nor do they strive after glory or worldly success; instead, they radiate their creative energy purely as divine-spiritual intelligence, as universal, divine love. This is the highest, most irresistible, all-penetrating power – the power of God. The sole activity of earthly prophets is to show the way to liberation and resurrection to those people who still dwell and suffer in the darkness or semi-twilight, and who are already fighting with all their might to escape from their suffering. These men are the servants of God. Most of them already have a vocation when they come into the world. But there have been, and will be, many others who attain this level only in the course of their lives. There have been, and still are, many such great men among us. In the West we call them saints, mystics, prophets, in the East, great masters, *rishis*. It is difficult to find them, for in appearance they are no different from other men, and they are recognized and understood only by those who are at *the level immediately below* their own. Others may worship them because they feel their greatness, but they cannot understand them. Some even hate them because they feel their greatness and imperviousness to all temptation, and therefore feel inferior and insignificant beside them. And yet he who seeks God from the depths of his heart finds these men, for 'by their fruits ye shall know them . . .' (Matt. 7:20).

At the seventh level man has developed his consciousness to such an extent that he is able to control all these forms of energy of creative-divine power *from the highest frequencies*, and can use them in each form without descending to the lower levels with his consciousness. He experiences life consciously within him, that is to say, in his consciousness he is life itself. In perfect self-recognition, in a divine state of self-awareness, in an absolute state of being, *in which not an atom of his being has remained unconscious*, he has become consciously identical, consciously one, with God. He understands, and can himself say what Moses said, because he too spoke face to face with God, that the name of God is: 'I AM THAT I AM'.

God is eternal *being*. And if in reality *I am* – the part of the verb 'to be' in the first person – thus, in my consciousness I have become *being* itself, God.

This is the very highest level of consciousness, at which man and his Creator cease to face each other as separate entities and the human Self becomes one with God in a monistic universal consciousness. Those who have attained this level, we call God-men.

That is why the God-man *best known* but *least understood* in the West, says of himself: 'I and my father are one' (John 10:30).

God-men live in a state of all-consciousness, of divine consciousness, and all their manifestations spring from this divine consciousness, from God *himself*. From time to time a God-man is born into this world to show that the attainment of this state of consciousness *is within everyone's grasp*. He shows us the path to God, to our heavenly FATHER, who awaits us in our unconscious, he shows us the path of the prodigal son, who one day awakes from the state in which he does no more than tend his bestial appetites, and says: 'I will arise and go to my father . . .' (Luke 15:18). And he comes to a decision and sets out on the long path of growing consciousness. He begins the great journey back to paradise, to the once deserted, heavenly home of the loving father, who comes towards him – us – with open arms, takes him – us – in his arms, presses him to his fatherly breast and in the sublime state of divine consciousness becomes *one* with him – with us.

# Chapter 9

# Saint George

Whoever practises Yoga in order to accelerate his progress on the great Jacob's ladder of growing consciousness must become thoroughly acquainted with sexual energy, which is the sole means of helping him from the lowest to the very highest step. He must make it completely conscious in himself and subjugate it to his spirit, that is to say, he must convert sexual energy into spiritual-creative energy.

As we have already seen, sexual energy, that universal force, is the creative principle – *logos* – and whether or not we are already aware of it, this energy is man's true being, his own Self, his own Creator himself, in the first person: '*I am it!*' For this reason sexual energy cannot be destroyed, since this would mean that man destroys himself. We can only transform sexual energy, only *be* it! And if a person has attained complete self-awareness with the help of this energy and has thus become his own master, he has also at the same time become master of sexual energy, the most magical of all magical powers, since *he is this energy itself*! The fully conscious man calls sexual energy 'I'. Such a man can work miracles and create new worlds around him with the sexual energy which he has converted into divine-creative power. He has obtained mastery over the whole realm of Nature with all her forces and all her creatures, he has become a white magician, a God-man.

The well-known representation of Saint George depicts this truth very vividly. The great saint, the all-conscious man, conquers the dragon – sexual energy – *but he does not slay him*, he merely pins him down with his sword. For *its fire and its strength are absolutely indispensable to him* if he is to reach God, if he is to *be* God. He must not destroy his own driving force, he merely subjugates it. For if he were to destroy the dragon, he would destroy himself and would no longer be able to heat his higher nerve and brain centres with the dragon's fire and radiate sexual energy as divine-creative power. If we wish to attain our goal – God – we are in dire need of sexual energy, subjugated to our ends and converted into creative power, in order *to use it as the driving force for spiritualization, release and resurrection!*

Those who have set out on the path of Yoga have usually a few steps from previous lives behind them and bear the experience, be it unconsciously, that the sexual energies may not be abused. They no longer wish to be caught in the snares of Nature, but to escape from them. But they too once had to acquire their experience of sexual energy, since the latter is equally God's manifestation of creative power, only, at the lowest level, the level of matter, manifested as spiritual power concentrated in matter, therefore as materialized spiritual power. If we spend this energy healthily, in accordance with the laws of Nature, this is not a sin. It only becomes so – if this concept is at all valid – when sexuality is abused for the purpose of dragging down the higher, spiritual energies by expending them without any inner harmony, as ends in themselves, in an exaggerated and unnatural way, through the glands stimulated by perversities and artificial means. This process robs man of both his will-power and suggestive power and greatly weakens his sexual organs. Everything that is performed by abnormally overstimulated organs in excess of normal, natural desires, as craving for pleasure as an end in itself, generally reduces man's vital energy, his mental powers and his character. On the other hand, he is entitled to expend sexuality in a healthy, normal manner. We know from the history of mankind down to the present day of many highly developed men who have possessed high spiritual powers and yet indulged energetically and with passion in the physical manifestation of love, without lowering and forfeiting their intellectual powers. They simply made proper and normal use of their creative energies in accordance with divine, natural laws. They experienced physical love and devotion based on healthy affection, therefore they expended *physical* energies *physically*. They did not transform spiritual, divine-creative energy into physical powers and use it in the opposite direction, nor did they drag it down to perversities and empty, purely sensual lust. At no time were they weak-willed sensualists at the mercy of sexuality.

On the contrary, they were masters of themselves and of sexual energy. Nevertheless, it is certain that however great they were, these geniuses who loved passionately were unable to become prophets, white magicians, saints and God-men, as long as they did not renounce their love-life. In spite of their human greatness, they were still identical with their sex, they were still human beings. Even if in the course of creative work they were elevated to the height of the divine spirit – which is sexless! – and during this time were identical with their genius, when the work was over, their consciousness sank again to a lower, human level, where they became sexual beings once more. In other words, they were not yet a *whole*, they were only on the way to becoming a *whole*.

A saint, a God-man has gathered all this experience in previous existences and Nature can no longer lure him into her trap. He has ceased to spend creative power through the sexual organs, but preserves it for his own body, without identifying himself with matter, with the body. He is conscious and remains so at the source of divine potency; he himself is this source as his own 'EGO' and no longer declines from this state of consciousness to the sexual, material level. Thus he directs the sublime, high frequency energies into his body, which is so completely transformed by them that the substance of the body of a saint or a God-man differs fundamentally from that of an average man. The spiritual powers destroy all bacteria and viruses, and so the initiated are immune against all illnesses. These powers preserve the body in a youthful condition, because the body cells are continuously regenerated by the high frequencies and high tension of the spirit. The hormones of the sexual glands are present not merely in order to endow the human body with the ability to procreate; instead they play a far greater part in the accumulation and preservation of youthful energies for their own body than is generally realized. Sexual energy is vital energy itself, the link between mind and matter. Not only can it transmit life in a *new* living creature during sexual union, but it can also continuously charge one's *own* body with new vitality, if one preserves it for oneself and knows the secret of its transformation. A saint, an initiate, does not despise the body, on the contrary, he esteems it highly as a wonderful agent of manifestation providing man with the only suitable driving force to climb the great ladder of Jacob. But since the initiate is conscious in his own divine Self – which is sexless – he requires no complement – whether physical or spiritual. In his consciousness he has become in every respect a *whole*. Thus he can preserve and use his vital energy for his own body, as he pleases, although his body continues to manifest quite normally and healthily one side of the whole, one sex, one pole.

As has been frequently emphasized, sexual energy is the link, the catalyst between mind and matter. If a man is unable to manifest sexual energy, if his organs of manifestation are missing or undeveloped, old or impaired, then he can no longer establish a direct link between his spirituality and his body – his spirituality and Nature. He can certainly attain the highest spiritual level in his consciousness, but he cannot transmit the magical power of the spirit to his body or to the body of other human beings. He can attain high spiritual awareness – this is possible even on one's death-bed – but he cannot acquire magical abilities, known as *siddhis*. He can become an illuminate, a saint, but not an initiate or a magician. There is no fire without fuel. There must be oil in the lamp when the bridegroom comes, the Bible tells us.

That should not, however, discourage readers who think they have already forfeited their sexual abilities. For man can never know when he has finally become impotent. We know of cases where old men who had considered themselves totally impotent for years suddenly experienced an unexpected resurgence of potency. And this is less exceptional than might be thought! On the other hand, we may ask the question: is it of such vital importance to each man to be able to regenerate his body, to become clairvoyant, to float above the earth and to acquire yet other magical-occult abilities? Is it not enough to be able to experience the highest states of consciousness, speak face to face with God in one's mind, live with an infinite peace in this world, and when time has run out on the cosmic clock, to depart this life? The fates of men are various! And each man must know himself what God wishes of him. If a person feels called upon by God to follow a certain path, he will then acquire all the possible means to find that path. Not only the laws of Nature, but also the divine laws are inflexible and insuperable. Everything depends on what we wish to achieve! For whatever we do *wish* to achieve – what our deepest conviction urges us to do – shows the measure of our maturity. Those who do not yet wish to give up their sex life, and those too who are sexually impotent, must take into account that, although they may indeed attain very high levels in the mind, the transformation of sexual energies into creative powers – that is to say, the expectation that they may become an initiate – must be reserved for some future life. At some time all men will reach the very highest, the divine level, and then they will also want no more than *to be* the divine *Self*, which is precisely what *all* this amounts to. But what we have not yet learned from experience and tasted to the full will always draw us back. For all that has not been experienced in man would have it so. Therefore do not let us resist, but let us try to experience as soon as possible, and leave behind us, all the things we have not yet experienced, if possible even before our 'individual source', 'the oil from the lamp' has dried up. And we ask ourselves: do we wish to remain slaves of matter, of the body, or do we wish to become master of the world of matter, of Nature, of our own bodies? Do we wish to attain the knowledge and power of the *'whole'* and enjoy eternal peace in God? Do we elect to go on being mortals or to arise and become 'living' people?

The divine laws seem inflexible to us only as long as we have not experienced them personally. If someone has the courage *to try out* these laws and possibilities *on himself*, and also *to live according to them* as a believer in God, then he will make the surprising discovery that these laws only appear to be 'inflexible' in the imagination of ignorant people. Man in his blindness is afraid of being at the mercy of these laws and of losing and missing something that – in his limited conscious being – seems of the utmost importance to him. He neither considers nor knows that this 'inflexible' God is *himself*, that in his unconscious he is the SELF that he calls 'God', but which in reality is his own, true, still unconscious being. Personal experience inevitably brings the great surprise that our true being, which as long as we are unconscious we call 'God', never takes anything away from us without affording us immeasurably greater happiness and joy in return!

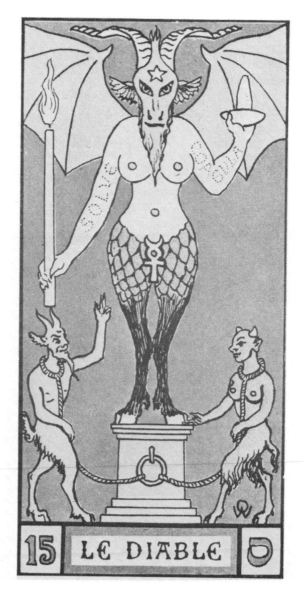

**15  LE DIABLE**

Satan is the law of matter which has come alive through the spirit. He separates the two sexes from each other – solve – in order to drive the two halves eternally together like slaves – coagula – without their being able to reach each other in the original divine unity. (Fifteenth tarot card.)

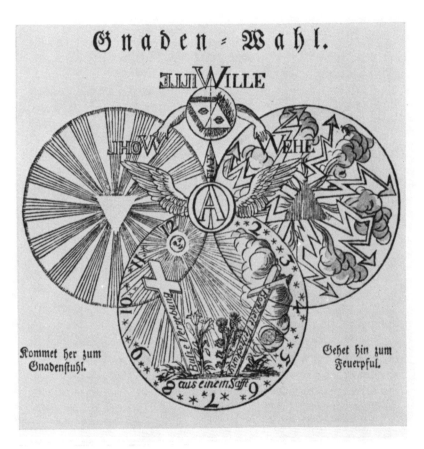

This was how the Rosicrucians depicted the twofold role and power of sexual energy: it leads either to the 'mercy-seat' – to divine self-awareness and bliss – or to the 'pit of fire' – to the decline of self-awareness, to spiritual gloom, fear and destruction.

# Chapter 10

# Urge for Unity and its Corruptions

God is eternal being – life – and God fills the whole universe. God, eternal being, life – where the two poles still rest within each other – is a unity which does not know duality. *Neither God, nor being, nor life is divisible.* This absolute, divine, single and unique unity is manifested in every living creature as its Self, which, in order to be manifested, has constructed the material form, the frame of the living creature, round itself and for itself. *Thus there is only one single, indivisible limitless, infinite Self:* God! And the innermost being of every living creature is this single, indivisible, divine *Self.* Paul the Apostle says: 'For God who commanded the light to shine out of darkness, *hath shined in our hearts* . . .' (II Cor. 4:6); 'For by *one* Spirit are we all baptized into one body . . .; and have been all *made to drink into one Spirit*' (I Cor. 12:13); 'And whether one member suffer, all the members suffer with it. . . . Now ye are the body of Christ [*logos*], and members in particular' (I Cor. 12:26, 27). In the language of today: the Self of God is the spirit and the whole creation, the visible universe, his body. We human beings are the cells of this gigantic body, capable of manifesting the sublime, just as the brain cells in our body manifest the sublime in our microcosmic being.

Every living creature therefore bears within him in his unconscious – where it is a whole – the unity of the Self, and this unity manifests itself in him through its unconscious urge to re-merge with the whole universe and all its living creatures and to become one with them. The Self, which requires the propagation of life for the spiritualization of matter, exploits this urge for unification, manifesting and fulfilling it in living creatures through the two great instincts: preservation of the self and preservation of the species. Both are therefore different manifestations of the urge for oneness.

In the first of these, the instinct of self-preservation, *logos* urges living creatures to become one with each other, in order to preserve life *in one and the same* material form – *in one and the same body*. In the second, the instinct for preservation of the species, living creatures are made to transmit life in *other*, subsequent living creatures, thus in other material forms, in *another body*, and thus to preserve the continuity of life in every possible way.

The instinct of self-preservation causes the larger living creatures to devour the smaller ones in their urge for oneness. Nature exploits this urge in order to nourish her creatures at the same time. Living creatures, however, feel this urge for unity even when they have no appetite. Anyone who has watched how a cat, *having caught several mice and therefore by no means hungry*, races after another mouse with passionate greed and devours it feverishly, only to vomit it again shortly afterwards, must certainly realize that behind the hunger and the gluttony a greater force, namely the urge for oneness, is at work. Living creatures have the urge to unite completely, to acquire an identity with others without sexual union. And since the mouth is the opening to the inside, they want to become one by the shortest way, hence they take their victim into their mouth, eat and swallow him. Animals yield to this urge and literally eat one another up. We human beings do the same thing, only we first cook or roast our victims. The tiger too yields to this urge when he races after the antelope and devours him, and all animals who bite into and devour one another do so out of the same unconscious desire for oneness. Human beings also know this urge, especially in cases where sexual intercourse is out of the question. The infant puts everything in its mouth although it is not hungry, and we adults say to a person of whom we are very fond, 'I love you so much that I'd like to eat you up.' And when one loves, one has the urge – which cannot be realized – to press the other person to one's bosom, to bite him, to force one's way into him. Unconscious urge for unity!

The instinct for preservation of the species causes living creatures to manifest the urge for oneness by imitating the unity of God, in which the two poles rest within each other, with the aid of the sexual organs.

There are also cases in Nature, where the urge for unity manifests itself through both these instincts, as for instance with the female spider and the praying mantis, which devour their mates immediately after sexual union.

How wisely has it been decreed that the urge to realize the unity of God compels living creatures through both instincts, on the one hand, to preserve life – to nourish the body, to eat – and on the other, to transmit life in new living creatures, to engender new life!

Since, in the divine-spiritual primal state, the two poles of creation, the positive and the negative, the giving and the taking, force and resistance, rest within each other in perfect equilibrium, there are, at the spiritual level, no separate male and female sexes, there is only the complementary unity of both. The spirit is one and complete in itself! Christ says in the Bible: 'The children of this world marry, and are given in marriage: But they which shall be accounted worthy to obtain that world, and the resurrection from the dead, neither marry, nor are given in marriage: Neither can they die any more: for they are equal unto the angels; and are the children of God, being the children of the resurrection' (Luke 20:34, 35, 36).

In the creation of the world of matter, the negative pole is expelled from the unity: thus they fall into duality and stand opposed as God and Lucifer, as force and resistance, as man and woman. But the unity between the two never ceases. It continues to manifest itself when they are separated, as tension drawing the poles towards and into each other. At the spiritual-divine level the poles fuse together and repose in each other, and physical-sexual union is the self-reflecting, imitating image of this divine unity. But fulfilment in the material body is impossible, for matter isolates, separates and keeps the two poles apart, in spite of the recurrent, desperate urge and attempt to attain true unity. The sexes try to unite, but fall apart again, and this occurs over and over again *ad infinitum*. A true unity at the level of matter is therefore impossible. Of all living creatures, however, man alone can *experience* the union of the poles *within himself as a purely spiritual state of consciousness*, although his body, if healthy, manifests only one sex in accordance with the present laws of Nature. For in the spirit the two poles have never separated, they rest within each other, and man bears this unity within him as *a state of consciousness, if he becomes conscious in the spirit.* The separation of the sexes exists therefore only at the level of matter, in the material, isolating world which offers resistance, in the body. The body manifests only one half of the wholeness of God and tries to reproduce the unity, not inwardly, as in the spirit, but outwardly, with an outside body, belonging to another being. Thus originates the creative, life-giving act of procreation.

The oldest playing-cards in the world, from which all other playing-cards derive – originally they were not 'playing' cards but part of the holy scriptures of the Jews, the cabbala, and represent the alphabet and the various levels of consciousness of man – this ancient tarot pack gives a witty and expressive depiction of this truth in its fifteenth card. Satan, the reflection of God – Christ calls him 'the prince', the law, 'of this world' (John 14:30) – who has become through the spirit the living law of matter, separates the two sexes (on his right arm is inscribed 'solve'), only then to reunite them with his left arm (which bears the inscription 'co-agula'); but not in their primal state, in the spirit, *inwardly*, but in the body, *outwardly.* The two sexes, male and female, which belong to each other by the inner unity of God, he chains outwardly together. Thus he forever drives the two sexes like slaves physically together, without their being able to reach each other in the original, divine unity. For the material outer world is the world of isolation, of separation, the world of good and evil, of giving and taking. To produce unity in the outer world is impossible. With our conscious minds we must step out of the finite, where our body belongs, and what we cannot do in the outer world, we *must seek, attain and experience in the inner world, in the mind, as a state of consciousness.* For only in our inner being, in our Self, which is God, can we spiritually find the complementary halves united in harmonious repose in each other. Man can unite the two poles *in his conscious mind.*

In the highest, spiritual state of consciousness, we experience the urge for inner, divine unity and its fulfilment as a very strange feeling. This feeling is not strange to average people, because they all know it and bear it within them, or do so because they at least desire to receive it from others. They have grown so accustomed to it that they take it as a matter of course and do not stop to consider that it is by no means so natural, but extremely odd. And those who have not yet made it conscious in themselves are for this reason incapable of understanding what and why it is! It has nothing whatsoever to do with the body. We call this feeling *love*. In order to prevent misunderstanding, let us call it *universal love*.

Naturally, every man conceives of this differently *according to his level of consciousness*. Regardless of this, if we wish to analyse what love is, we could speak of it roughly in these terms: we have a pleasant, warm sensation in our hearts. It cannot be measured with a thermometer, and yet we feel it as 'warmth'. We radiate this warmth quite involuntarily. These rays are invisible, immeasurable and their existence admits no proof, yet we feel this radiation of love from ourselves, as from other creatures, so distinctly that no one can deny it. It radiates spontaneously, and under its effect we have the desire to unite our being with the whole universe or with something that we 'love'. We know the expression: 'I am so happy that I'd like to hug the whole world!' It is an urge for unity *without physical reaction*. This feeling has nothing to do with sexual desire, nothing whatsoever to do with the body, for we certainly have no sensual-sexual desire towards the whole wide world, and yet the feeling is there: a purely spiritual feeling, a purely spiritual state. One would like to melt into the universe, to be absorbed by it, to become one with it as a raindrop becomes one with the ocean when it falls into it. *Only the superior man* who has activated his higher nerve and brain centres and can therefore sustain purely spiritual high frequencies, is capable of this purely spiritual love. The inferior man with his undeveloped consciousness projects divine love into the body and makes of it a sexual attraction. He is not yet able to bear spiritual frequencies, nor therefore comprehend them with his intellect. Hence the spiritual level does not show what a man *knows* – for one can have a brilliant intellect without a high spiritual level; nor does this level depend on whether a person is charitable, for one can be charitable with one's intellect by outwardly imitating a person who is full of love. The spiritual level manifests itself *in the wealth of love a person bears within him*!

That is why Paul says:

Though I speak with the tongues of men and of angels, and have not charity, I am become as sounding brass, or a tinkling cymbal. And though I have the gift of prophecy, and understand all mysteries, and all knowledge; and though I have all faith, so that I could remove mountains, and have not charity, I am nothing. And though I bestow all my goods to feed the poor, and though I give my body to be burned, and have not charity it profiteth me nothing. (I Cor. 13:1, 2, 3.)

With people at the lowest, still unconscious level, the urge for unity of the Self is also manifested. Since, however, their consciousness is still identical with the body, the urge manifests itself in the great, corrupting fallacy of wanting to experience and manifest spiritual unity, the urge to merge with the whole world, in the body. They want to offer their body to anyone with whom there is a possibility of physical union, and they do so indiscriminately. A very sad consequence of this is that these people – who basically are also looking for love, if in quite the wrong way – degrade themselves, give up, lose their human dignity and prostitute themselves. The laws of the spirit are opposed to the laws of matter, of the body. If, therefore, the laws of the spirit are divine at the spiritual level, then, at the level of matter, manifested through the body, they are satanic. The reverse is also true: the laws of matter, manifested through the spirit, are also satanic. Paul says: 'For the flesh lusteth against the Spirit, and the Spirit against the flesh: and these are contrary the one to the other: so that ye cannot do the things that ye would' (Gal. 5:17).

It is understandable that prostitutes the world over are despised by those people whose consciousness is *slightly* more developed. Those labelled here as prostitutes, include not only the official prostitutes, for among these are very often people whose degradation is due to indescribable poverty. For our purposes, prostitutes are those who offer themselves more or less indiscriminately to anyone, without the pressure of destitution. Anyone who has once had a heart to heart talk with prostitutes – male or female – must have witnessed their sad feeling of neglect, worthlessness and hopeless ruin, their utter despair and self-contempt. When asked why they go on with such a life, they almost invariably give the desperate reply: 'I am looking for a little love.' These poor souls do not realize that it is precisely what they are doing which makes them betray the very love they are seeking, betray their own Christ with a 'kiss', they expend love, lift up their heels against it, kill it, because their deed does not spring from an inner harmony which binds two people together. It is particularly sad in the case of women, who should guide their husbands on the long path to God, to divine consciousness. God says to the serpent: 'And I will put enmity between thy seed and her seed; it shall bruise thy head . . . (Gen. 3:15).

A person of a very low level of development, who experiences physical union as a mere sexual discharge, devoid of any inner affection, selection or feeling of spiritual love towards his or her partner, sooner or later falls prey to dreadful fear and emptiness. Unconscious people do not know how very deep a bond sexual union creates between man and woman. They each absorb a part of the invisible being of the other. We have only to think of how a person can irradiate and charge a lifeless space, a room, the compartment of a train or a theatre stage with his presence, so that it is felt long after he has left. He leaves his radiation behind and thus charges the walls, pieces of furniture or perhaps the armchair in which he sat, in such a way that a dog for instance, but also sensitive people, recognize and feel his radiation long after he has left the room. How much more powerful the mutual influence of people who experience sexual intercourse with each other! How frequently we can observe the way in which people, through persisting in a sexual relationship with a partner unsuited to them, gradually change, transform their own nature, their character, often for the worse, sometimes also for the better, and acquire certain qualities of their partner. If two people share their love-life, or even if they have had only a single sexual encounter, they are mutually affected by vast invisible forces, for sexual energy is creative, it is man himself! And however strong a person's conviction that the powers and radiation of an 'uninteresting' or 'insignificant' being – as one often hears – have no effect on him, these nevertheless leave an imprint, the depth of which he does not suspect.

In Dante Alighieri's masterpiece, the *Divine Comedy*, this truth is aptly depicted: in one section of Hell Dante sees a multitude of souls which have grown together in couples, flying around in despair, in untold suffering, because all their most strenuous efforts to separate from each other are in vain. During their mortal life they were bound only by physical love relationships, not however by true love and togetherness. Animal passions for their own sake and crude sensuality were the cause of their encounter. Therefore they are now inseparably and eternally bound together by their own defiled, spiritual aura, and also by the continued, inextinguishable memory of their deed.

The sullying of man's invisible being, however, does not result only from his experience of sexual intercourse with inferior beings. It will also occur whenever people who are not necessarily bad, characterless or impure, but simply ignorant, have sexual intercourse with *a large number* of partners, indiscriminately and at random, today with one, tomorrow with another. We can put the most beautiful colours on a palette, and yet we obtain a hopeless mess if we mix them *all* together. The once beautiful colours lose their character completely and are no longer recognizable. Therefore we can understand why prostitutes all have their typically hopeless, impure radiation, why they have completely lost their individual, human character, so that they are recognized from afar as prostitutes.

It is even more tragic when young girls of decent, good families degrade themselves out of sheer ignorance and boredom by having sexual intercourse indiscriminately with the first chance comer whose acquaintance they have just made, and a day or a week later repeat this with a second, then a third or a fourth.

How much patience, trouble and love, and how much time is required before the bad impressions, all the impurities and the dreadful inferiority complex are removed from such a broken young soul and self-respect is re-established! And anyone who has not had the chance of observing these circumstances for himself would simply not believe that the partners, male or female, through whom these desperate people feel lowered and neglected on account of their sexual experiences together, have taken away with them the same degrading impressions. *It was therefore not one person who degraded another, as neither of them was an unclean being, but the sexual intercourse as such, which they experienced indiscriminately and devoid of love.*

Contemporary civilized life is so degenerate that men no longer have the opportunity to achieve something heroic, entirely on their own merit, which would allow them to have a sense of their own worth, to 'feel great'. Young people go into a cinema and watch enraptured how the great cowboy or detective excels and triumphs over all the others with his superhuman abilities, while they themselves have no chance of accomplishing heroic deeds and of displaying their own outstanding abilities. What remains for them? For some, the answer is sport. For the great mass of young people, however, there remains nothing else but to assert themselves through sexual conquests, and thereby to experience higher tensions. Out of boredom, out of a hopeless feeling of emptiness and thwarted achievement, they are driven to sexual experiences and other addictions. Thus they have a mutually defiling and degrading effect on one another. Most of them are unwilling to admit this profound effect, because they are unable to recognize what takes place not in their conscious mind but in their unconscious. Because their conscious mind is not aware of and does not experience a phenomenon, they refuse to believe that it nevertheless concerns them, that in spite of their unawareness, something has happened to them. And precisely because it has taken place in the unconscious, the effect is a thousand times greater than if they had been able to digest it in their conscious mind. In the unconscious, things remain undigested and therefore often have a poisonous effect on men. Nevertheless, people feel, even if unconsciously, the poisonous effect of sexual intercourse with an unworthy partner, and try to protect themselves by instinctively leaving the whole matter to the body, and withdrawing the conscious mind 'as much as possible' during sexual intercourse of a degrading nature. In this way a person cannot experience healthy and gratifying fulfilment, even physically, simply because he is not totally involved! And the consequences are mental and physical disturbances which can lead to apparent impotence.

*Mind, soul and body are an indissoluble entity.* For as long as man lives, they cannot be separated from one another. The body comes last: it is the manifestation of the spirit which is furthest removed in the scale of creation, but it is nevertheless part of it, it has grown together with the mind, and they consequently form a unit. It is a great mistake to believe that the mind can experience a thing without the participation of the body, without the body sharing the experience – and vice versa; everything that happens to the body reacts upon the mind, the mind shares the experience, *since it is the mind which builds the body, vitalizes it and experiences everything in and through the body itself.* Without the mind the body is an inanimate corpse. Consequently, everything that happens to the body is felt and experienced only in a man's mind, in his Self, in his consciousness. If consciousness is switched off – as for instance during narcosis – man has no perception whatsoever of what is happening to his body and what his body is experiencing. Therefore there are no separate physical *and* mental experiences and perceptions, there are *only* mental experiences! And this is true even if these experiences project themselves into the body. *We experience only what our consciousness – which is purely mental – perceives.*

It is the same with our sexual experiences: however convinced a person may be that he accomplishes and experiences sexual union only out of purely physical desire, it is nevertheless impossible for his experience to be *purely* physical, for the 'experience' in itself is possible *only* in the mind, *only* in consciousness. In the case of a woman it may happen that *only* her body participates in a sexual union – of course completely passively – that is, if she is drugged or anaesthetized. With a man, however, this is unimaginable. And with a woman, such a case cannot be regarded as 'participation' or 'experience'.

If, in physical union, a person tries to withhold his mind, because his sexual act does not manifest itself and grow out of spiritual oneness, then a split, a gap, occurs in his being, whether or not he knows or acknowledges it. Conscious men feel this and refrain from such physical release. Unconscious men, however, imagine that they can have sexual union out of *purely* physical needs, without involvement of their mind. And that is a great mistake. For, regardless of whether a man has been gratified or frustrated, if he is secretly worried about, or even ashamed of his behaviour, he has already participated in the union. For 'being frustrated', 'ashamed', or 'worried' are also inner states of consciousness, but not physical reactions. Sexual energy is man's being which manifests itself in the body – *logos* itself. And so it is also impossible to want to experience sexual union without the true Self. It need be explained no further that man can only speak of true, physical joy, of physical fulfilment and the sexual happiness of lovers, if physical oneness grows out of true love, true spiritual harmony, and he can abandon his whole being to the feeling of sexual happiness without subsequently having to feel shame.

The primitive man is content with any partner of the opposite sex who physically answers his simple taste. He attaches no importance to a 'spiritual' inner union, since he himself is not yet spiritual, awake and conscious. But a man with more developed consciousness, with more pronounced individuality, can experience the real joy of love and true gratification – physically and spiritually – only with one partner, who above all harmonizes with him in spirit, *and reciprocates love of every kind with love.*

We only feel at ease in shoes and clothes which have been made to our personal measurements. This is *really* a purely physical matter, and yet it has an influence on one's whole state of mind. How much more important it is that a man finds the partner who is suited to him *in every respect*, in mind, soul and body, who is in every way his complement, whom he *can* really *love*, in whom he *can* really *trust*!

As we have seen, it is frequently the case that young people as well as adults engage in sexual intercourse with the first person who comes along; this leads to man's making an animal of himself. *But man is not an animal!* Let us not forget that. These words are not the product of sentimental or religious false morality, but of the experience acquired over three decades with a very large number of young people and also adults, who in their mental and physical distress sought help and have continued to do so in an ever-increasing number. The West, too, has discovered that sexual repressions can give rise to serious mental and physical disturbances. Consequently, the pendulum has swung to the left, and many people want to rectify all mental disturbances by giving free rein to sexual desires – whether real or imaginary – without moderation or discrimination, and by trying to overcome inhibitions, which have often a purely psychic cause, with sexual excess. But the time is near when the pendulum will again swing to the other side, and men will be led back from artificially bred animality to a clean humanity. Many despairing people return from a dead-end, from a total abnegation of life, indeed even from the urge to commit suicide, to normal life, through *an uplifted way of thinking and way of life.* Misguided people mistakenly believe and teach that the one and only salvation from the different forms of mental distress is to lead a licentious, sexual life and to squander one's energy indiscriminately. But men seek love – and they seek it also in sexuality, even if erroneously. Anxiety and existential problems can never be solved by sexuality.

# Chapter 11

# The Sun – Creator and Destroyer of Life

If a practitioner of Yoga feels the need to lead an abstemious life in order to make faster progress on the path, then he should first examine himself thoroughly to find out whether he – or she – is mature enough for this. He should not act like the fox who finds the grapes too sour because he cannot reach them and therefore does not want to eat any. He should be ready and able to digest higher nourishment because he has eaten so many of the 'grapes' that he knows them and does not need any more. He can be given advice on how to live abstemiously without incurring danger. For an abstemious way of life only makes sense if it is *profitable* and not harmful.

At this point it is again necessary to speak of patience. For it takes time to activate the higher nerve centres through a completely continent life. Nor can one make an adult of a child if its time has not yet come, and if one were nevertheless to take away its toys and compel it to behave like an adult, it would still not grow into an adult but would become mentally ill. Thus we must wait patiently until the higher nerve centres indicate that they are becoming active, and that the transformation of sexual energy into higher forms of energy has become possible. This does not happen overnight. Therefore, if we have reached the stage where we feel sufficiently mature to lead an abstemious life, and we arrange our life and practise accordingly, we must even then not be impatient and expect higher results immediately. We may be satisfied if initially there appears a striking love of life, cheerfulness, a bright suggestive shine in the eyes and increased working energy.

Our long experience shows that with those who are mature enough, living abstemiously can generate and accumulate so much vital energy that, if it is applied in the right way and directed consciously, chronic illnesses which have lasted for years are suddenly cured and serious neurasthenic symptoms disappear. The posture becomes youthful and elastic, the mind grows bright and clear, even severe depressions disappear. The power of concentration increases in unsuspected measure, one begins to acquire the power of suggestion, the body is filled with new vitality. We have often been able to witness that through abstinence, white-haired practitioners of Yoga have regained their original hair colour, that shrinkage of the gums and other symptoms of old age, which nowadays occur too early in men, have disappeared, and some could even read again without spectacles.

If a man transforms sexual energy in the right way, he can be sure that in the course of time, sooner or later, higher spiritual benefits will not fail to accrue. Man suddenly discovers talents which he never in the least suspected within him. They were already present, as they are in every person, but still in a latent condition. If we erect a dam in front of the sexual energies, they then accumulate, initially causing tensions and unrest. If, in spite of this, we stand firm, these energies look for new paths and we become capable of gradually converting them into higher powers. Sexual energy that has been directed upwards first of all stimulates the secretion glands, thus renewing and strengthening the body, then stimulates the higher nerve centres, which until now were only capable of manifesting potentially present creative powers as different talents. That is to say, the nerve centres which would have been capable of manifesting these talents lacked up to that point the corresponding resistance and were in a latent condition. How often we come across historical cases of men who, after a dissolute way of life, suddenly for some reason or other began, or were forced to begin, to lead an abstemious life, and shortly afterwards manifested outstanding talents, in particular an exceptionally strong magical-suggestive power, the existence of which no one, least of all they themselves, suspected. We may mention here only the instance of Ignatius Loyola, the founder of the Jesuit order, who, as the result of an accident, had to lie for some time in his father's castle, and out of sheer boredom experimented with secret exercises because he was forced to lead an abstemious life. In the course of these experiments he made such unexpected discoveries that he completely altered his conduct; together with friends he founded the Jesuit order and in the space of fifteen years acquired power over the whole world – as far as China! He himself claimed to have achieved his renowned magical-hypnotic will-power through an abstemious way of life and *secret exercises.*

At this point it is again necessary to note that an average man can only grow into a superior being in possession of magical-suggestive powers by leading an abstemious life, if he has progressed so far in experience, development and maturity that he is able to sustain and endure the irritation of the retained sexual energies on the higher nerve and brain centres *with calm nerves, imperturbed and without pathological irritability.* The best support in achieving this can be gained from some particularly appropriate Yoga exercises to be discussed at length.

If a person is still insufficiently mature for a transformation of sexual energies, that is to say, *if his higher valves have not yet been opened* and his consciousness is therefore still very limited, and if, in spite of this, he is forced to lead an abstemious life for any reason – be it a physical, congenital abnormality, disturbance or anything else of that nature – then he will fall ill. Usually, over-strain first affects the thyroid gland, which may cause heart disorders, but inevitably causes an intolerable flight of ideas, anxiety states and still other, more serious disturbances. In such cases the roused sexual energy does not find a valve for itself. Nor does it find the way to the higher centres through which it could manifest itself as higher, spiritual energy, and it causes pathologically excessive irritation, which involves very great danger for the nerves, because it is continuously inflamed from within. This danger may cause a serious nervous breakdown, indeed it may even give rise to a yet more dangerous condition, which in modern terminology is known as 'schizophrenia'. Anyone who has had the opportunity of studying schizophrenic patients in a mental home must have noticed that almost all of them without exception have experienced some obstacles or disturbances – no matter whether of mental or physical origin – in expending their sexual energies, and that they very often possess an astonishing intellectual level and high abilities. They often have insight into the highest spiritual realms and glimpse very high spiritual truths, while, on the other hand, they are still undeveloped, unequal to this high intellectual level and unable to withstand, digest, or adapt themselves to the high tension of superior intellectuality. They cannot make any use of it, and their nerves cannot sustain this high tension, this split condition, since they have no opportunity for release. There is an undeniable connection between manic attacks and the frustration of sexual energy. A person who deals with the mentally ill and who himself leads an abstemious life – therefore having the benefit of personal experiences and observations – has no difficulty in understanding the condition of these patients. Unfortunately, however, these observations are not all that is needed to help them, even though the insight is of the clearest. My reason for referring to these illnesses in the course of this discussion lies elsewhere. The work with these patients produced a strange discovery: most of them had not *intentionally* withheld from sexual life, on the contrary, they would have liked very much to lead a sensual-lecherous, perverse and licentious life, if they had not been prevented from doing so by physical or psychic reasons. Now certain of these patients who were intelligent enough to understand the truth about sexual energy, went as far as using their sexual inhibitions, *quite consciously and deliberately*, to lead an abstemious life, for the sake of transforming this energy. *In these cases there was quite a marked improvement in their condition*, which gradually led to their becoming able-bodied, useful members of society. The voluntary abstinence of these patients had to be coupled with the change to a morally superior mentality. They had to be led back to God! This is not so easy to achieve with such patients and therefore in only a few instances was an improvement possible. But *those* cases where there was such a vast improvement that one could really speak of a cure prove the deep link between schizophrenia and the sexual energies *unintentionally and involuntarily* dammed up. They also show the possibility of recovery through belief in God, or at least through a morally cleansed mentality together with *deliberate* abstinence, in which case there can be no question of repression – since the process is a conscious one. On the other hand, we have never seen a cure attributable to unrestrained and indiscriminate enjoyment of sexuality, only decline and ruin!

A man can only be helped by himself, for one cannot intrude into another person's consciousness and put it into order. At most we can indicate the path that leads to it – *if we ourselves know this path*! Alas, it appears time and time again that most of those who want

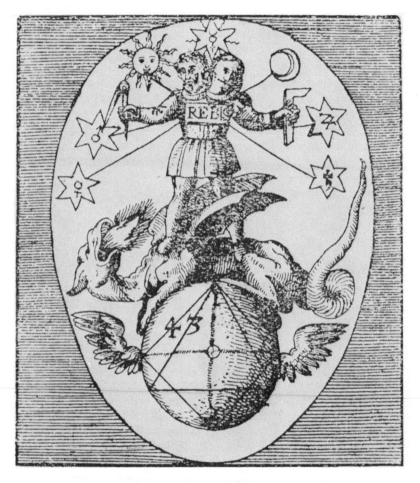

The Rosicrucians called a man who attained all-consciousness, thus
making the two poles conscious within him, a 'hermaphrodite' – composed
of Hermes and Aphrodite – and depicted him with two heads. He is
master of sexual energy, of the dragon, the 'lord of this world'; he stands
on the dragon, who in turn rules the earth. The all-conscious man uses
the dragon's fire to stimulate and keep active his higher nerve and brain
centres.

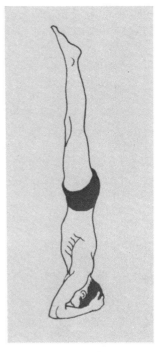

Headstand

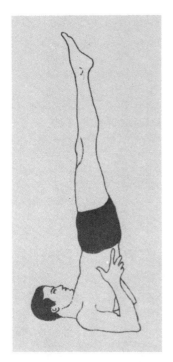

Candle Posture

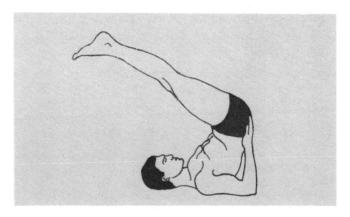

Shoulderstand

to help these patients are themselves still very far *from having recognized* creative energy in each of its manifestations *in themselves, and from being able to direct its course.* This just cannot be learned at a university or from a book, *but only from personal experience!* One rarely finds a professional psychologist or psychiatrist who has experimented with sexual-creative energy in himself and acquired his own experience. *If a certain period of abstinence was prescribed, purely as an experiment, at universities, Western psychiatry would be plagued by fewer misconceptions!*

Experienced sportsmen have long since discovered that we can store a great amount of energy through abstinence. Competitors are forbidden for a minimal period of six weeks to drink alcohol, to smoke or have sexual intercourse. It would be *highly instructive* to introduce such periods of abstinence into the study of medicine and particularly of psychiatry so as to provide personal experience.

However incredible it may seem, the following incident is true: we were acquainted with a very well-known and distinguished doctor. After he and his excellent wife had brought five handsome sons into the world, he chose to adopt an abstemious way of life, which, in his own words, allowed him to preserve all his energies and to concentrate much more on his patients, to achieve much higher accuracy in his diagnoses and to find instinctively the best method of curing his patients. And his attractive, healthy and highly intelligent wife was in complete and loving agreement with her husband, who felt nothing but charity for his fellow-men. Such things do occur and, thank God, not just as rare exceptions.

The Bible says:

> For there are some eunuchs, which were so born from their mother's womb: and there are some eunuchs, which were made eunuchs of men: and there be eunuchs, which have made themselves eunuchs for the kingdom of heaven's sake. He that is able to receive it, let him receive it. (Matt. 19:12.)

All this had to be said in order to explain why a person who has taken the trouble to gather his own experience, not from theory but practice, will always say here or in the East that an abstemious life is not suitable for everyone but only for spiritually mature men, to whom it brings beneficial results. Such a man has realized how one can direct the creative powers upwards or downwards and use them as one pleases. But he has also realized the dangers involved in the transformation of sexual energy. If a person is firmly resolved and is afraid of nothing, then he may attempt the process. But even then, he may do so only if he does not endanger a marriage partner who is not yet mature enough for this. This remark is certainly not intended to frighten off those people who wish to progress on the divine path of Yoga. For we have in our hand the best weapon against all dangers: our own consciousness! If we always cling to it, that is to say, if we are always awake, if we are always conscious *here and now*, then no harm can come to us!

Infinitely more dangerous than the attempt to lead an abstemious life, are certain Yoga exercises affecting the spinal cord which at the present time are propagated by ignorant and unscrupulous men. For against the danger involved in abstinence there is the very simplest protection, namely, to give it up immediately, should it be the cause of discomforts such as pathological nervousness or excessive irritation. We must realize that creative energy is no trifle, and that these matters are to be taken quite seriously. Those of us who have had the opportunity of repeated investigations in convents and monasteries know what sad consequences may ensue if immature men and women are forced to renounce sexuality and sacrifice 'all'. As long as we regard that as a sacrifice, we are not mature enough to make it. God demands no sacrifices of men. They are very, very few indeed who have already acquired spiritual maturity and can transform sexual energy into divine-creative power. Many are the 'called' and few the 'chosen'! But the chosen have existed and will always exist, in the monasteries as well as outside, throughout the whole world, here as in the Orient! Therefore let us progress with courage on our path!

# Chapter 12

# The Magic Flower

There is really no point in *talking* about transforming sexual energy, because mere *words* are to no avail. It has to be *done*! In doing it we gain personal experience and all words on the subject become superfluous. Therefore we can *say* very little, but if this 'little' is put into *action*, it becomes everything!

For what is meant by the transformation of sexual energy into spiritual-creative power? To use sexual energy as the link between spirit and body, not in order to create matter from spirit – to beget children – but, on the contrary, *to obtain spiritual energies from the body*. *Not* to spend sexual energy through the body but, instead, to open the higher centres through which it manifests itself no longer as sexual energy but as spiritual and creative-magical energy. How do we open these centres? Through control of the body with the exercises of Hatha Yoga, by mental concentration and meditation, abstinence and work! That is really all that needs to be said.

Yet, we shall try to say a few guiding words in answer to the numerous questions posed by our practitioners of Yoga with reference to this subject. We are aware that not all questions can be answered satisfactorily. Since the subject touches on very delicate matters, it is not possible to speak frankly about all the relevant details. In this case only one thing can help the practitioner of Yoga: to acquire his own experience! What surprising discoveries we make then, which not only answer all questions instructively but also bring us experiences hitherto unimagined and unexpected. Experience will then reveal to us further secrets which have always been latent in man – and the human body – while we have remained unaware of their possibility, that is of their existing in reality and not only symbolically. We shall therefore attempt to describe the first steps on this path and also how to advance on it. The further, higher steps, however, will be deliberately only touched upon. Those who take this path seriously and practise will themselves see the continuation of the path before them, and will know how to proceed, just as a person holding his small lamp before him in the darkness sees where to take his next step.

Those, on the other hand, who are only prompted by curiosity to know these things, but do not make the effort to do something, do not require to know even theoretically how, and by what means, man can unshackle and employ his creative powers – powers inherent in all men. That there have always been, and still are today, powerful magicians – let us call them what we will – the greatest of sceptics cannot deny. We therefore try to hand on the key to the door of the secret chamber, but each man must open the door himself. What treasures will be found there, and how they are to be used – there is no need to say more about that. Each man will know himself, without further explanations. . . .

If we wish to climb up Jacob's ladder, we must above all have one thing, without which there is no progress, and that is *patience*! The spirit, the Self, is above time. The spirit is timeless. Patience is the state of timelessness. Hence, if our goal is to awaken spiritually and achieve spiritual consciousness, we must first of all adjust our minds to timelessness. And if the devil of impatience tries to take hold of us, we must at once console ourselves with the thought: in eternity there is time enough! Just as a Chinese or Indian painter never works on his timeless masterpieces while thinking: 'I must hurry to get this finished on time' – otherwise he could never accomplish these breathtaking works of art – so, too, must the practitioner of Yoga renounce all notion of time with regard to his inner progress. Even if, by using the method for quickening the growth of his consciousness, man shortens the way to divine self-awareness by thousands of years, this process of development takes time. Eternity is long enough and God knows exactly how much time we require to follow our path to the goal. We do not need to worry about time. Only the person lives in time, in the finite; our spirit – which is the spirit of God – does not know time and space. Let us do everything to shorten this way as much as possible, but let us never think of how much time we shall take to do so. This thought would paralyse us and make us feel the lashes of time on our back. The spirit is timeless, and whenever we think of time we crucify our own spirit, our own Self. That is why we become so nervous if we have to rush, if others hurry us on impatiently. For the Self – Christ-*logos* – is crucified on the two great beams of time and space, and if we do that with our own Self – with our own Christ – we lose the strength and courage of the spirit which we so sorely need.

The fact that he does not notice his own progress is the greatest test for a practitioner of Yoga. Just as a child does not perceive when he grows into an adult, so a man does not notice – or only rarely so – when his consciousness expands, rises and he becomes more aware. Just as someone who gets into a lift on the ground-floor, locks himself in and ascends, does not notice what height he has reached, since he was always *'there'*, *with himself* in the small cage, and can only estimate it when he gets out at the top and looks down, so the practitioner of Yoga does not notice when his consciousness expands and how many rungs he has already left behind him on the great Jacob's ladder. Only if he now and then casts a backward glance, does he see what ignorance and darkness, compared with his present state, he has emerged from.

Therefore we must not be impatient, for each moment is precious and affords us a new, interesting experience, however uninteresting and boring it may seem at the time. Everything, each experience, however small, helps us along the path. There are no relapses, at most, apparent relapses. People who have trod the long path before us, who have reached the goal and want to help us, describe the landmarks of progress to us and the milestones we must leave behind us one by one. They also describe *how we can leave them behind us*! Just as in the lift we are helped by the number on the wall sliding past, which shows us the floor we have reached, so, with the help of the masters who have gone before us, can we ascertain which step we have reached. We recognize the milestones and can proceed on our way with courage and hope, and when we have reached the summit of the mountain and have a strong foothold, we can help those climbing up behind us.

An accelerated development – whether of flowers or of the human consciousness – always involves certain dangers, because, after all, it is not the way of Nature. *These dangers can, however, be avoided, if we know them and arm ourselves against them from the outset.* One can ascend the steepest rock-faces to the summit of the mountain provided that one is properly equipped and knows where particular care is required. Many people conquer the mountain with an experienced guide; others, again, like the first conquerors, reach the summit without a guide. But *once* they have got there, they are both equally *at the top*! Therefore we must know the dangers of a quickened transformation of our sexual energies, and learn how to proceed in safety from the example of our precursors.

By far the best, and the surest weapon against danger of any kind, is *never to lose hold of one's consciousness*. That is to say, that the consciousness must always be identical with itself, *here and now*, that it must not drift away and become identical with external things. *We must hold on to our own consciousness, never let it go*, therefore we must always be *awake*, always *here*! The consciousness is the magic flower which leads the prince on the path to the top of the mountain where his bride lives, and which saves him from all the dangers of darkness, threatening him in the form of evil spirits and gnomes, but also of enchanting fairies who want to lure him on wrong paths. He holds the magic flower before him and the supernatural light which it radiates shields him from the evil spirits, the gnomes and dangerous fairies, chases them away and lights up the path so that the prince cannot lose his way. *The light of the magic flower is our consciousness!* We must constantly examine our every feeling and thought and penetrate each one with the light of our consciousness. We must notice the slightest stirring of our soul, of our mind, and immediately examine its source and its unconscious motive. The mask concealing many an urge, many a feeling which arises from the unconscious, but which we do not wish to acknowledge, must be relentlessly torn down. There are dangers which disguise themselves as our benefactors, which dress up in the guise of sublime faith or piety. Let us find out what lies behind this. How often are errant sexual desires, sensuality and perversities hidden under the mask of charity, of so-called altruism, or even under the guise of the highest religious ecstasy and ostensible mysticism. We must know that the higher a person's consciousness rises, the simpler, more modest and temperate, more *awake* and *calm* he becomes. But let us beware: our simplicity and modesty should not be a part to be played, a put-on show. If a person *wants* to be simple and modest, he is still far from actually being simple and modest. Feelings and waves of emotion indicate the wrong path! What is outside is not inside! How often do we find falsely 'pious' faces and gestures masking the most vulgar personal vanity. This shows the desire to be acknowledged already as a selfless 'saint' – and particularly important – *to be ranked higher than other, 'ordinary' mortals*. The higher we are in our consciousness, the more natural and simple we become. Not because we play the part, but because *we are as we are*! We already understand and know why Christ replied to the young man who addressed him as 'Good Master': 'Why callest thou me good? There is none good but one, that is God' (Matt. 19:16, 17). If, then, a person has a *good* thought or word, or does a good deed, then God is in that person, manifesting himself through him as that which is 'good'. The superior man is never complacent and arrogant, because he is not puffed up. He is never amazed at his own 'greatness' and 'goodness'; he finds it natural that he has these qualities, and never thinks of himself as 'great' and 'charitable'. In his consciousness he has ceased to be the superficial mask, the person, he has become the *core*! And if a person is conscious all the time, his inner eyes will open and for him the 'two sides of the tree of knowledge of good and evil' will fuse together. For him, concepts such as 'good' and 'evil' will cease to exist. He sees only the tree, which is *one*. He no longer knows anything that is good or evil. Such words denote appearances only. The illuminate, however, sees through appearances; for him, such differences disappear. There is nothing that is 'good' or 'evil', there are only the manifestations of God, which are all good; only if unconscious men use and expend them wrongly, by mistake or out of ignorance, do they appear to be 'evil'. Everything is *good*, only in use can a thing become satanic. There are no ill powers, only powers put to ill-use! 'Nothing is good or bad, but thinking makes it so' (*Hamlet* II:2).

If we are continuously on the alert, if we do not permit ourselves the slightest emotional stirring without being conscious of it, repression or any other harmful effect of an abstemious life will be prevented.

# Chapter 13

# Practice

The transformation of sexual energy is quite easy, and for that very reason may seem difficult to some. One is reminded of the anecdote about the apprentice alchemist who had received the infallible formula for making gold and proceeded to try it out. The most important requirement was that on no account should he think of a hippopotamus while preparing and boiling the mixture. The following morning, when asked by his master how he had got on, he answered thoroughly depressed: 'I followed all the instructions and did everything correctly, and it would have been all right. But now, although I had never known before what . . . a hippopotamus was, when I was not supposed to think about it, a whole herd raced round in my head. And so my mixture did not turn into gold!'

Provided that the disciple's mind is in a constant state of time-lessness – patience – then our first advice on this path is that the disciple, who is moved by inner conviction to lead an abstemious life, must on no account whatever make a vow! For if someone believes that he is really mature already, that he will never again think of sexual desires, that he has risen above them and that his body obeys him, and he then takes a vow, the Devil will seize him immediately and strike terror into him. He will believe that 'all' has now been irrevocably lost. Henceforth he will – he must – think continuously of his vow, he will be unable to think of anything else, whether he wants to or not, as if all the devils had been let loose and descended upon him. These devils are nothing else but 'the animal in us' as Paracelsus called this power of the body or, 'the flesh lusteth against the Spirit . . . so that ye cannot do the things that ye would' (Gal. 5:17), as Paul described this power. And since the thoughts are turned to sexuality again and again, the sexual organs are irritated, and the candidate will keep having sexual desires and sexual fantasies. All at once he will understand St Anthony in the Sahara Desert who for forty years continuously saw highly erotic scenes, naked women tempting him and so forth, and had to fight these visions. Of course, 'the devils' conjured up these images for him. Today we should say that his 'unconscious' projected them, but the result is the same – it is only a question of designation. Finally, after forty years, St Anthony did manage to conquer the devils. But in vain! For behold, they are still alive today, they have even increased in number and all descend upon the poor ascetic who has made a vow.

The making of vows is therefore *not* advised!

*Once more, however, we recommend* that one should give up abstinence and lead a sex life based on true love if intolerable torments have to be fought against. That is neither a disgrace nor a sin. In this way too progress can be made, albeit more slowly.

If, however, anyone perseveres in order to reach the higher stages as quickly as possible, our advice to him is that he should completely *forget* the vow and every possibility of one, and at the same time also *whatever* his vow was. He should *totally forget* sexuality and all that is connected with it. Very simple, isn't it? If only the devils did not exist! For, even if we have seen through Nature's deception completely, and find the whole business of sex with its eternal repetition very boring, the surest formula for unbearable sexual desires which suddenly spring up and rouse the corresponding physical reactions, is for the intellect to be preoccupied with sexuality, which we really wish to conquer. Thus we learn how the negative pole manifests itself and acts on us from our unconscious as the *spirit of resistance*. It is not surprising that in religion it is called the Devil. And it is not so easy to deal with this "Devil, since I am it. I AM IT, taught in the Upanishads as: Tet Tvam Asi, Tat Tvam Asi,— Thou art that."

Apart from the devil of the unconscious, the body itself for the time being allows us no peace. Until now the body has been adjusted to a sexual life, the glands continue to demand release, and as long as sexual energy does not find the way to the higher centres of manifestation, it accumulates in the sexual glands. Later, when sexual energy *has found the way to the higher nerve centres* through appropriate Yoga exercises, *and can manifest itself there already* as a higher form of creative power, the transformation is much easier. Then one also has much more peace. The initial period is the most difficult, precisely because sexual energy, *unable to find an exit*, irritates the sexual organs even more. Thus, at the outset, man has a twofold difficulty to overcome: on the one hand, his imagination, his intellect allows him no peace, on the other hand, the retained sexual energy stimulates him physically still more than before. *But that is exactly what is needed!* For this excessive stimulation gradually reflects upon the higher nerve centres, irritates them, and this irritation wakens them from their latent, dormant condition, as the prince wakens the Sleeping Beauty with his 'kiss' ('kiss' being a sexual manifestation). If one has therefore struggled through the first difficulties, if one has resisted and overcome the mental and physical irritation, then the transformation is very much easier – by way of reward. It is also very important, however, that we allow the upsurging sexual energy to manifest itself through the higher nerve centres, to pour out through them. What is our best help here?

*Yoga exercises, concentration, meditation and work!* Physical and intellectual *work!*

The first of the Yoga exercises is pranayama, that is to say, control of breathing.

We can only really grasp the importance of breath control if we realize the fact that every sexual union imitates breathing, that is to say, the rhythmical union of the breath with the lungs. Every breath we draw is an act as life-giving as the encounter of the sexes. Breathing gives us renewed life with every breath, while sexual union gives life to a new being. That is why correct breathing gives a fulfilling, pleasurable sensation akin to that of sexual union.

Pranayama and the physical exercises – known to the Indians as Hatha Yoga – serve to invigorate and spiritualize the body in general, thereby, of course, making and keeping it healthy. These exercises have been described in detail in the book *Yoga and Health* which I have published together with my colleague, Selvarajan Yesudian. The present book is really a sequel. Hence, I shall mention here only the Yoga exercises which are particularly suitable for those practising abstinence. These exercises make the blood flow from the lower to the upper part of the body and the head, thereby calming the sexual organs and rousing the higher centres. Then follow descriptions of the special exercises for the transformation of sexual energy into spiritual energy, and of the exercise which enables us to control and use vital energy as animating, magical fire.

### CANDLE POSTURE (SARVANGASANA)

The effect of this exercise is to bring the blood from the legs and abdomen into the head, the brain centres, neck and shoulders. We thereby strengthen the organs of the brain, which are the source of our memory and power of concentration. We also strengthen the thyroid gland which has its seat in the neck, which directs our intellect and heart and provides our sense of time. Thus pressure on the heart is reduced and its activity regulated by counterbalance.

*Technique*: lying on the back, we press our arms extended parallel to the body with the palms facing downwards on the ground. We breathe out calmly and deeply, and slowly and carefully raise the stretched legs until they are vertical. Then we raise the trunk, supported by both hands in the kidney area, until it is in a straight line with the feet. We breathe with the stomach and hold this position until strain is felt. Then we return slowly, first with the trunk and stretched legs, and lie for a few moments on the floor breathing quietly and regularly, which restores the blood circulation to its normal course. In performing the exercise there must be no abrupt and jerky movements, which may damage the heart.

### SHOULDER STAND (VIPARITA KARANI)

The effect of this exercise is similar to that of the Candle Posture, but the execution is simpler.

*Technique*: lying on the back, hands parallel to the body, we breathe out and slowly raise the legs. Supporting the hips with the hands the legs are brought down slantwise behind the head. In this the exercise differs from the Candle Posture. Also, the hips and not the trunk are supported by the hands. Breathing calmly with the stomach we hold this position for as long as possible without strain. Then we return slowly and controlled to the lying position and calm ourselves with gentle, and at the same time, controlled breathing.

### HEADSTAND (Sirshasana)

The effect is similar to that of the Candle Posture, but the highest brain centres, in a latent, dormant condition in the average man, are more powerfully affected. These centres are activated through the exercise (also through complementary exercises in concentration). We thereby gain access to the consciousness of the creative power within us, our memory is stimulated and higher mental powers awakened.

*Technique :* in the starting position we kneel on the ground and sit on the heels. The hands are cupped with the backs to the ground. Then the head is bent down and approximately the upper crown placed in the cupped hands. The elbows are on the ground, pointing not too far out from the body. Now the trunk is raised and the legs stretched. When we have found our balance we raise and straighten both legs until they are vertical. We may raise first one leg, then the other, or both together. The position is held, with regular and calm breathing, for as long as possible without undue strain.

This posture occasionally presents initial difficulties. If this is so, we begin the exercise in the corner of a room or in front of a divan, which allows the raised, vertical legs some support if necessary.

In returning to the starting position we bend the legs and proceed to the kneeling position, sitting on the heels. In this way we experience a sense of peace for a few moments. On no account may we fall out of the headstand or make other abrupt movements.

### TRANSMUTATION (OJAS)

This exercise is the most important and most effective for the transformation of sexual energy. I sit in Padmasana (Lotus Posture), breathe with perfect Yogi-breathing, and with activated imagination I visualize that *I myself* – therefore my consciousness, my spiritual Ego – descend to the coccyx with every inhalation, and from there with slow exhalation ascend in the spine, that is to say, in full self-awareness I slowly ascend to the skull which is the seat of the Sahasrara *chakra*. The description of this exercise is quite simple, and yet it enables us to deflect all irritation away from the sexual glands to the higher centres where we can store sexual energy as creative power – provided that we do this exercise correctly. It is therefore the most important transformation exercise of all, for it helps us to *conduct* sexual energy upwards to the higher centres in order to manifest and use it through these centres in its converted form as creative-magical power.

Our first task must be, with the help of sexual energy, to increase the resistance of the organs, in which until now creative power has lain dormant. The resistance must be raised to a level which allows creative power to emerge from its latent condition and become active. It *no longer* manifests itself as sexual energy, but as spiritual – magical power. Progress then depends on learning the next exercise: to conduct the spiritual power, which *I myself am*, everywhere in my body, that is to say, to penetrate everywhere with my Ego, and to send my radiation into my whole body. For it is not sufficient to transform sexual energy, my own materialized Self, and at the same time to conduct it up to the higher centres, but rather, with the help of these same higher centres, our highest goal is to radiate and use vital energy as magical power. It is not enough to make the philosopher's stone. We must know *how* and *to what purpose* it can be used. Otherwise it is useless to possess a magic wand; if we cannot *use* it, then we are not magicians.

This exercise is really very simple. It amounts to *redirecting the consciousness* in a way which enlists the aid of creative-magical power, thus becoming a magical and vitalizing act. What has made it take on these qualities? – The fact that *I myself* have consciously become this power. *The 'I' is life, and where I consciously* AM *there is also* LIFE. *Wherever I consciously penetrate, everything becomes vital and life-giving.* Anyone who considers these two sentences and understands them correctly knows all the secrets of life and death.

The technique of the exercise is as follows: with the perfect breath control of Yoga we take a very deep breath and inhale deliberately to the apices of the lungs. Then, with the exhalation – which must be slow and somewhat withheld – we direct our consciousness first to the tips of the feet, that is to say, *I myself go there with my Ego*. We shall feel distinctly how a current is generated in the feet, as well as an initial warmth, which, later, when we are more practised, becomes a fiery heat, a hot prickling sensation.

We practise in this way for about five to ten minutes at the beginning, later prolonging the period, for under no circumstances can exercise be harmful. We need not look at the clock. During the exercise we shall know exactly when our concentration gradually begins to fail and we can then stop.

Without perfect concentration, that is to say, if we are not totally involved, there is absolutely no point to the exercise. The best position for performing it is lying on the back so that the blood can circulate evenly in the body. In time, one can feel the feet being charged with the higher frequencies of concentrated consciousness, and a tingling warmth gradually rising in the body. Accordingly we can then raise our consciousness together with the irradiation, and charge the legs with higher vital energy. Then we can begin to irradiate the hands, first the right, then the left and then both simultaneously, until they too feel the warmth and prickling. We can extend the process to the whole trunk, to the body, so that we have a general feeling of enhanced vitality as of tingling warmth, even as of heat. In the whole body we become awake! The body receives this radiation like an open vessel and begins to *live* much more intensely. The whole body from top to toe, to the tips of the fingers begins to live and be awake everywhere with such intensity and vitality that one feels it is filled with light, with intense rays of light.

This is more than just a sensation. It indicates the fact that with this exercise we develop an ethereal body woven of light. Some mystics call this invisible luminary 'diamond body'. The Bible describes it in the Gospels. Christ appeared to his three disciples on the Tabor mountain in his 'transfigured body': 'And after six days Jesus taketh Peter, James, and John his brother, and bringeth them up into a high mountain apart. And was transfigured before them: and his face did shine as the sun, and his raiment was white as the light' (Matt. 17:1-8). 'And his raiment became shining, exceeding white as snow; so as no fuller on earth can white them' (Mark 9:2-3).

Just as we can make a piece of 'dead' metal magnetic – alive – by means of electricity or another magnet, so through this exercise can we make the human body magnetic, alive. Just as magnetism is a magical power, so the human body becomes capable of manifesting and emitting human-magical powers and energies. Thus we attain mastery over the magical-creative energies. It is true that this can only be achieved with transformed sexual energy.

Just as sexual energy can give life to a new living creature, to a child, so this life-giving energy can create a new living creature *in us*, can direct the vital energy of a new living creature into our own body. Thus the old mortal 'Adam' becomes the new, resurrected and immortal 'Christ-man'. From the energy of the higher, enhanced consciousness grows an increased vitality, whose high frequencies tolerate no bacteria, no viruses. This explains the immunity of God-men to all illness. Even if one has not yet become a God-man, one can already use the extra powers of increased consciousness, according to the individual level, at first, then in a modest way, then in an ever higher and more spiritual manner.

If there is a disorder anywhere in the body, we can focus this irradiation with full intensity on that place. And we shall discover with astonishment that, through the focused vital energy, pains disappear – often quite suddenly – and catarrh and other physical disorders are cured. The frequencies of consciousness are incomparably higher than the so-called short-waves, X-rays or radium rays. Naturally the effect, too, is incomparably greater.

We can produce miraculous effects not only in our own body, but, if we are skilled in the direction of consciousness, we can guide these high frequencies also into other living creatures. In so doing we establish order in their bodies. At this point one hesitates to go on. If we consider how mischievously these matters are abused by ignorant, inferior vain people, then we understand why it is better to keep silence. Great magicians such as Mesmer, du Potet, Marquis, Puységur and others have spoken frankly on the subject. The inevitable outcome, then as now, is that ignorant people start playing with these powers. Usually out of vanity, they want to aggressively 'magnetize' others *who have no desire for that whatsoever*. In so doing they transmit their own impure radiation to other suffering people, who, as a result, then become really ill or worse than they had been before. Therefore let us restrict our ambition to acquiring increased vitality for ourselves, and learning to direct and use it properly. Let us make our bodies alive and – awake!

A person who does these exercises *out of true desire for God* will have inner experiences of such a novel kind, so many hidden doors will be opened to him, that, sooner or later, out of real love – and

127

not in order to be admired – he will want, and indeed will be able, to help others. At this level he no longer needs to learn from other people how and to what purpose his own, higher radiations can be used and applied. Nor did Ignatius Loyola, Father Barré or Valentin Greatrakes learn from anyone how to cure maniacs and other seriously ill people. That is why we shall not pursue the subject.

Let us therefore practise with an iron will, and the key to the transformation of sexual energy into creative-divine powers will be placed in our hands.

However, I should like to repeat one piece of advice. During the Yoga exercises we should never think that we are practising because we wish to still our sexual glands in order to be able to lead an abstemious life. For the Devil never sleeps, and if we turn our thoughts to the sexual organs, they are irritated and roused by the direction of consciousness. Therefore, when we practise Yoga, let us think of health, peace and balance, but in particular let us try to awaken, experience, and put into practice, the sense of *wholeness*. Let us try to experience within, the sense of perfect independence. Let us arouse in ourselves the assurance that in no respect do we require a complement, need help from outside, *expect* love from others, but that we *give*, that we have and are everything – *everything* – within us. *I am a WHOLE!*

This feeling gives us unshakeable self-confidence, fearlessness and courage! It becomes a state of being which we constantly have within us. We are always content, because we have everything within. This state helps most of all against any sexual desires. *For sexual desire stems from a feeling of deficiency, from the search for a complementary half which we lack, without which we feel alone and forsaken.* If, however, we have found *everything* in ourselves, if we are a *whole*, what more do we require? What can we lack?

The general beneficial effect of the Hatha Yoga exercises can be further reinforced by physical activity. In the same way as the Hatha Yoga exercises, physical work helps us to direct our thoughts and the excess blood-flow away from the sexual organs. Sexual energy is the vital energy which man can retain for his body. A good means of achieving this is physical work together with the performance of Yoga exercises. Work not only occupies the body and distributes the blood evenly through the muscles, but also engages the intellect, thereby preventing the thoughts from wandering off in the wrong direction. Apart from their spiritual pursuits, monks and nuns work in the fruit and vegetable garden or in the various workshops of the monastery. We can do other kinds of physical work or go in for sport. However, it may happen in the course of purely physical activity that the intellect repeatedly slips off in the wrong direction, while we are hoeing potatoes, rowing, playing tennis or whatever we may be doing. We are tempted again and again to think that the purpose of our work is to direct the sexual energies into new channels so that the flow of blood to the sexual organs is prevented. This in turn directs all the thoughts, the whole consciousness, and as a result, the entire blood-flow, to these very organs. Strange to say, already from these first struggles we gain the very useful experience that it is not the body that causes sexual desire, not the body that disturbs us, but the intellect! Against this it might be argued that sexual desire influences the intellect from the unconscious. Granted – but only till such time as sexual energy finds the way to the higher centres. For if one has progressed so far in one's own experience that transformed sexual energy can be manifested as creative power, then it is no longer repressed into the subconscious and no longer acts from there like a poison. Even then if one wishes, sexual energy can be conducted back to the sexual organs and expended as sexual energy, *with the help of the intellect*. The intellect is capable of turning the steering-wheel wherever the consciousness commands. And already at the start of our struggle with the creative energies we realize the magnitude of the task the intellect has to perform on our way to God. How blessed is this serpent which by its 'coiling' not only leads our vital energy downwards, but equally also upwards, to God – if our consciousness is master over it!

We are well aware that in puberty the body makes itself felt with elemental force. The vital tension is high and the sexual energy very powerful. That is why the young *adolescent*, if he controls his sexual energy and converts it into spiritual-creative power, can *make the quickest progress on the spiritual path and attain to God!* A young person has the fuel richest in calories to stimulate the higher centres! We see, however, that with sexually powerful animals, sexuality plays a much smaller part in their life than with those people who with the help of the intellect frequently increase and augment their sexual reactions. The unsuspected importance of one's mental attitude with regard to the sexual glands is shown by experiences people have had in situations of danger.

After the siege of Budapest in 1945 many men and women who had witnessed this terrible blood-bath became impotent through unutterable fear of death. How did the sexual organs know that the person carried the fear of death in his consciousness! How does the genital organ of each man and animal know that progeny must not be begotten in time of mortal danger? Natural scientists are very familiar with the high wisdom of Nature which manifests itself in disasters. Fear of death in Budapest caused many women to miss a period and men to become impotent. On the other hand, we know the case of a man whom a female enemy soldier wanted to seduce by force, and since he showed no desire whatsoever, she tried to compel him at the point of a gun. The man, who at that time was very alarmed at the apparent total loss of his potency – he had been impotent for some time – suddenly, out of pure fear of death when threatened with the revolver, in spite of his dislike of the strange aggressive woman, became capable of gratifying her desire. In this case fear of death had exactly the opposite effect, it restored potency.

We could list further instances which prove how a person's mentality affects the sexual organs, and thus the sexual desires too. But the way in which Nature can react with resistance – the basic principle of homoeopathy – is shown by another case. A man who had been impotent for years determined at least to exploit this condition in order to become 'holy', since he had to lead an 'abstemious' life in any case. Curiously enough, the moment he made this decision, his body reacted by manifesting hitherto unsuspected potency! Therefore in this case, too, the obstacle was not presented by the body, but by the mentality, the cast of mind.

*Thus at the very outset of abstemious life we discover, quite consciously, the unimaginably effective power of the intellect and thought!* And with that we have made the first great discovery and experienced it personally. The first, the most difficult step of all has been taken!

We can, therefore, with the help of physical work deflect the energies from the sexual organs, but this is only effective if by a parallel process we then divert, silence the arch-enemy – the primal serpent: the intellect, our thoughts – and keep on doing this until we have gained mastery over sexual energy. The best way to achieve this is to occupy the intellect with something else. 'Two things cannot be in one and the same place at the same time', therefore, we must expel all sexual thoughts from the intellect by replacing them *with thoughts of a different kind*. We have said that an abstemious life should not be embarked upon as long as sexual desire does not fall away itself like a ripe fruit from a tree. The question now arises: if a struggle is still necessary, why should we engage in it at all?

Firstly: There is no such things as a 'should', a 'must'. We give this advice only to those who wish to practise Yoga in order to make the fastest possible progress, because they feel in themselves *the insatiable desire for God*. One thing, however, we must not forget: anyone who has progressed so far in his inner being that, out of *conviction*, he wishes to renounce sexuality and use sexual energy merely as fuel for the stimulation of his higher nerve and brain centres (a rough comparison would be the warming of radio valves by electric current) still has 'an animal in himself' as Paracelsus puts it. Even then that person has a body and in it the glands which were previously used for regular sexual gratification. Since the glands are unable to understand why their possessor suddenly wishes to engage in abstinence, they continue to demand release from the tension caused by accumulated sexual energy. Nature, however, is very elastic! And in the same way as the glands have grown used to regular release, one can gradually get them out of this habit with the help of the consciously controlled intellect and of appropriate Yoga exercises. Of course it takes time, longer in some cases than others, until the person – of whatever sex – is able to adapt his glands and assert his will also in the body. He will learn in the process how to liberate himself from the bondage of the body and be master in his own house. He will be aided by the closely linked spiritual and physical Yoga exercises which we have mentioned before, and by – *creative activity*. For we can only open the higher centres *if we give them the chance to emanate creative power*.

The exercises which help us in the transformation of our energies are chiefly of a spiritual nature. The physical exercises are of help in conducting creative power *up* to the higher centres; the spiritual ones, on the other hand, in *using* creative power. We must learn how to control the thoughts and the intellect and how to direct them where we wish. We must learn *to think about what it is we want to think about* and not about the random subjects which our thoughts introduce to the mind and compel us to reflect on. How much this is discussed and how few are those, even among ardent practitioners of Yoga, who take the trouble to try and put it into practice! Most people expect the physical Yoga exercises to improve their concentration without *their own inner effort*. Exactly the opposite is true: we can only perform the physical Yoga exercises properly and effectively if we focus all our attention on directing our concentration inwards. *The only possible way to learn concentration of thought is precisely by concentrating. There are no magical charms which allow lazy people to concentrate without their own inner effort!* Through physical Yoga exercises we can increase the supply of blood to the brain centres thus making them more powerful and vital, therefore able to obey and serve us better. The brain centres, however, can only obey if there is something there to command and use them properly. And once more this 'something' is nothing other than ourselves! Who and what else? Let us therefore command our brain centres, send a great amount of energy to the brain and think what we want to think and in the manner we want to think of it, *not as the thoughts themselves suggest.* For this we can take the converted sexual energy, which we have not expended but retained for ourselves. Of course the power of concentration can also be increased and high spiritual levels attained without an abstemious way of life. But we get incomparably faster results, and a noticeably stronger effect, if we retain the fire of life for ourselves. Sexual energy is a form of manifestation of *my own Self* – I am it, even if unconsciously so. We shall therefore understand that if I do not expend sexual energy – therefore myself – through the body, but preserve it in and for *myself*, I strengthen *myself*, therefore my *will-power* and my *magical, suggestive radiation.* I can therefore greatly increase my ability to be *myself.*

We must strengthen our hold on the body. If the glands are irritated and project sexual fantasies and desires on the screen of the consciousness, then we do not let ourselves go, but ask ourselves: 'Who is stronger: I or the sexual desire of my body? I am of course!' and we immediately occupy ourselves very intensively with something else that attracts our attention. We have learned that two things can never be in the same place at the same time, and we push all sexual thoughts out of the intellect with other thoughts. And – here is the surprise – the body obeys and sexual desires are silent. Whether we then go for a walk and watch the birds flying, whether we go fishing and concentrate until a fish bites, whether we stay at home and practise Yoga or read an interesting book, whether we play the piano or another musical instrument, whether we do gardening or train our dog or quite simply attend to our daily work . . . it is entirely up to the individual. No two people have the same interests, no two people have the same fate. Each and every one must and can feel in himself where his talent, inclination and chance lie, and what interests him so intensely as to make him forget sexual desires. It makes no difference how we divert our attention from sexual desire, the main thing is *that we divert it!*

How does the body react at this level? As long as we are completely absorbed in creative activity, the body does not react at all. It enjoys being charged with higher frequencies whereby it becomes healthier and shares in the illumined state of the EGO. It may happen that, on completion of a continuous piece of work followed by a few days' rest, the body announces itself, at first by erotic dreams during sleep, and then also when we are awake. Obviously, we are therefore not yet at the level where we are always consciously able to direct the body, that is to say, the current of life. Thus we continue to practise the special Yoga exercises and start working again with all our strength and concentration.

If someone can use his energies in creative work and still has insuperable difficulties with his body, we advise him to pacify his body with a normal sex life. Indeed the body desires sexual gratification much less frequently than is imagined by those people who do not leave their glands in peace, but rouse them with highly spiced food, stimulant drinks, erotic reading matter, films and other such excitants. This only overtaxes the glands, weakens them prematurely and condemns them to ageing. Animals illustrate how rarely Nature desires sexual intercourse.

Everything depends on *what* we desire. Desire is the supreme power and it takes us exactly where we wish to go – where we wish to go *with our whole being!* In this connection we advise one thing in particular: to refrain from praying to God for HIS help in overcoming the sexual urge. Let us not forget that God dwells in us, behind our human consciousness in the great *unconscious*, and HE himself – God – wants to advance our progress along the path of development. Therefore HE helps us in any case – usually HE even forces us – much more than the unconscious man suspects, for God *himself wishes to become conscious in us and through us.*

However, in order to pray to God to remove our sexual desires (which, alas, many people do quite apart from the fact that such a thing is childish) we again concentrate on sexuality, turn the intellect afresh to the sexual organs – and hell is let loose! Let us not beg God to help us overcome our sexual desires, let us, rather, *help ourselves!* Anyone who wishes to attain the supreme, divine stage and whose yearning for God is so intense and profound that he is interested in nothing else, will be led by his strong desire to the path on which he can turn away from sexual thoughts and desires without torment and devote himself with calm nerves to the transformation of his energies without begging for help. If, however, someone who is already at a higher level now and then yields to his sexual urge, that is neither a disgrace nor a sin! He is still a human being of flesh and blood and no one has forbidden him to enjoy his sexuality. And precisely for that reason he must not make a vow at the beginning of his path, so that there will be no cause for shame should he once nevertheless yield to his sexual desires: shame, not because he has enjoyed his sexuality, but because he has *broken his vow.* What is past cannot be helped, and if he has once had physical union with his loved one, honourably, out of true love, with inner devotion and healthy physical desire, he must on no account regard himself as a weak, fallen and sinful man. Why should he? God has erected no barriers before us and does not lay down that we *must* lead an abstemious life. Therefore do not let us dictate to ourselves, but ask ourselves, what it is we want to have. And if the desire for freedom is greater than the power of the body, then *whatever we do is done of our own accord!*

And so, we continue to practise. One day we shall succeed in calming the glands through constant diversion of our thoughts and they will trouble us no further. We can continue our journey along the path of spiritual development. As far as men are concerned, this point is a new test. For men feel, even if unconsciously, that sexual energy is of much greater significance for their own being than is the procreation of a new generation. Deep down in themselves they feel that sexual energy *is* man's being. That explains why men – already in childhood – protect their sexual organ, which they identify with sexual energy, with painstaking care and shield it from all possible danger. They have the feeling, and quite correctly, that something irrevocable, terrible would happen if they were to lose the organ of their virility, and with it their potency. The male feels instinctively that *through the loss of his sexual energy in its material manifestation, he himself* would be destroyed.

The following characteristic incident may illustrate and help us to understand this test: we had a very valuable, spiritually superior friend, who had become a monk in order to be able to devote his whole life consciously and sincerely to the search for God. He was a powerful and spirited man. Night after night he could not sleep at all because his body allowed him no peace. He did everything which might have helped him but the Devil had apparently not yet done with him. One day our friend came to us obviously in despair: 'Just think,' he said, 'suddenly I can sleep very well, I can concentrate on my work undisturbed, my body has stopped reacting, it does not bother me at all. Goodness me, do you think I have become impotent?' I had to laugh aloud: 'Listen,' I said to him, 'for a long time you have been practising with a great deal of effort to calm your glands so that you can freely devote yourself to your spiritual progress. And now that your efforts to lead sexual energy to higher centres have been crowned with success, are you alarmed that you have succeeded in what you so earnestly sought and wished for? Don't worry, you have not become impotent. On the contrary. You have come near to becoming the source of all potency.'

Man is like that – even such a resolute, strong character as our friend the monk! These are the 'children's ailments' which man has to come through before he has gained experience if he has not been born as one already 'anointed' or 'chosen'. And there is no disgrace in getting these ailments. 'Strait is the gate, and narrow is the way which leadeth unto life. . . .' (Matt. 7:14), said Christ, and he knew what he was talking about. He too struggled for the kingdom of heaven and fasted in the desert for forty days, and just when he changed from Jesus of Nazareth into Christ, the Devil's temptation was stronger than ever. Naturally, the 'Devil' does not spare us either, but we must remember this great example and know that *victory is possible*!

Of course, even then if we have reached the stage where our glands do not trouble us, it may happen that, for instance, if there is a south wind, they reawake and project erotic thoughts in us. In that case, we practise the Yoga exercises and continue to occupy ourselves with physical and mental activity, all of which repeatedly and ever more effectively helps and calms us. Even if the doors to the higher centres have opened for sexual energy, for a time it still flows back to its lowest exit of manifestation where it acts as physical-sexual energy. The old path, once made broad and easy, still lures and draws the current of life to itself.

The next step affords us already much greater joy. Our struggle is no longer solely to calm the sexual organs and to gain control of our thoughts, but rather we begin to use the sexual energies directed away from the sexual organs, transformed, *as spiritual powers*. The first great step has been taken – the doors, hitherto closed, to the higher centres of manifestation have been opened. How can we now apply these spiritual powers?

This reminds us of the great wisdom spoken by an owl to the magician in a Walt Disney film. The magician wants to explain to a child which feathers a bird uses in order to rise off the ground, and which he uses to keep his wings moving in the air. The owl listens for a while and then says, irritated and full of contempt: 'Fancy trying to explain about *learning* to fly. One learns to fly simply by *flying*!' How wise, how true! One learns also to transform sexual energy simply by transforming it. Let us be quite clear about this: what is meant by transforming sexual energies into spiritual powers? Is there an apparatus in men where the vibrations, the frequencies of the energies can be transformed and changed into different forms of manifestations? Yes. There are several. They are the *chakras* which not only send out rays, but also function as transformers. We know this, however, only with our intellect. If I use the nerve centres, the seat of the *chakras*, I experience the various vibrations not as 'vibration' or 'frequency', but directly as conscious states of being. I take as an example the ears, that is to say, the auditory nerves which receive all the vibrations of sound and impart these to my consciousness. Although I have learned with my intellect that the sounds are vibrations and that the different sounds have different frequencies, my consciousness will not perceive them as different vibrations, but I shall *hear* them quite simply as different *sounds*. I shall be unable to notice the number of vibrations, more or less, of one sound compared with another, but, I shall *hear* them as *lower-* and *higher-pitched* sounds. So it is with creative power. In its lower vibrations I shall be unable to notice how they *vibrate*, but rather I shall feel and notice them *in my body* as sexual urge. In its higher vibrations – in my soul – I shall feel them as love, as the spiritual urge for unity. Even higher, as the urge for creative manifestation, as natural talents, as intuition and creative ideas. In their very highest frequencies, I shall *be* them, as a purely spiritual state of being – as I AM.

Just as the ears and auditory nerves enable me to hear sounds, so that I am aware of the sounds but not the ears and auditory nerves, so I am aware of creative power with the various organs of manifestation and the *chakras* as the sexual urge, as feelings and as direct states of being. I feel the activation of the higher nerve and brain centres only to the extent that I suddenly become intuitive, that I have creative ideas and an inclination for creative work, that unsuspected talents come to light, that there is a remarkable increase in my will-power and power of concentration, that I become self-assured and I notice by my effect on other people that I have acquired suggestive powers and as a result have become the centre of attention. Therefore I must not expect that the *chakras* and their seat, the higher nerve and brain centres, announce themselves by any kind of feelings or other signs, when they go into action. I notice the ears, auditory nerves and other sense organs, as also the higher nerve and brain centres and the *chakras*, only if they are not quite in order and perhaps cause pain. As long as they function healthily I am not aware of their existence.

I shall be as unable to gauge the frequency differences as – to remain with our example – the ears are to gauge the vibration differences of sounds; they transmit them to my consciousness as lower or higher pitched sounds, which I then simply hear.

It is only as various states of consciousness that I can feel directly, experience, or in the highest form, become identical with the various frequency differences of the various forms of creative power. And if I call these forms of manifestation *lower* or *higher*, I do so for the same reason that I call a sound *lower* or *higher* because I *hear* it *like that* – lower or higher! If we explain what a sound is, then we can give as detailed a description as possible of the vibrations and frequencies of sounds, and yet we shall be totally unable to make a creature that has no ears understand how we hear a sound, or indeed, what it even means to *hear*. I should be still less able to explain that a sound may be 'lower' or 'higher', and least of all what the difference in sound is, for instance, of a flute, a violin or an organ. If this creature once tried to hear – and managed to do so – then it would *hear* from personal experience, instantaneously, directly and without need of further explanation.

A further example: we cannot explain the taste of a chestnut to someone who has never eaten chestnuts even if we were able to give a perfect scientific description of the frequencies of this taste, or even write books on the subject. That person will have no idea of the taste of chestnuts until such time as he tastes one himself All that is going on and all that is stored in our brain is only *outside* and is not a *conscious state of being*. I *am not* identical with it. The taste of the chestnut will only become a conscious state of being when we taste it with the tongue and experience it. The tongue and all the other sense organs can transmit their perceptions to me as a state of consciousness; *the brain, the intellect can never do that*. We see how difficult it is to give explanations about the transformation of the creative powers. It is absolutely futile to explain rationally. *We can only know* the nature of things *through direct experience*. I can *experience* nothing through the intellect, precisely because it is incapable of *being* anything. Once we have understood these matters correctly and wish to experience them, we must transmit them from our intellect to our being, as a state of being, and through our direct knowledge, experience *being identical* with them. We shall then learn to become ourselves the taste of the chestnut when we taste it and experience its taste within us.

Explanations about the transformation of sexual energy can only be given in as much as one shows how to *do* it. All these things will then be *directly experienced* and *understood*. As long as we do not make the effort, we shall never be able to understand the nature of *the bliss, fulfilment, absolute contentment and self-confidence* which we experience as a conscious state of being if we have become able to transform creative power from its sexual form into its higher form, and can say, *I am it*. How can a mineral solution know and apprehend what is happening when it is crystallizing? The molecules automatically fall into a crystalline lattice, which only this mineral solution can produce, because *it is it*!

Thus each one of us will only be able to be *what* he is, and that cannot be explained in advance, because each person is an individual manifestation of God, and is therefore different from the next person. Just as the mineral solution began to do something and could do nothing else but become – *be* – itself, its own characteristic Self, and manifest its being in a crystallized form, so we, too, must *do* something, and we shall be unable to do anything else but *become ourselves and manifest ourselves in crystallized form*. In this way we shall experience the secret of creative power directly and understand it through BEING. Only those who already understand it because they *are* it, can give advice. Each one of us must learn to *be* through his own experience.

How do we begin? With intellectual, creative work. And with what work? Let us not ask that. We shall in any case only be able to do *what we are*. And what we want to do is what we are. We shall do, then, something for which we have a talent and an inclination, and pursue it according to the time at our disposal beyond our normal working hours. For so many men, so many fates, so many paths.

To those men or women who have their regular jobs, which scarcely leave them time to further their progress on the spiritual path, we recommend the practice of meditation during a quiet time of the day.[1] If anyone has begun to lead an abstemious life, he will notice that meditation is infinitely easier than before. It has already been explained that retained sexual energy accumulates, vital tension increases and this heightened tension acts on the spine as a strong irritation, as a powerful stimulus. Thus the higher nerve and brain centres are automatically heated, roused and activated like the valves of a radio. This state is manifested in man's consciousness by his becoming *more awake*. He begins to *live*! Only now does he notice that hitherto he has hardly lived. He did not live, he merely vegetated, his life was a farce. He breathed, ate and drank, even worked, but he always had the feeling that he did not participate in life – that he had no share in it – everything seemed to him like a

[1] cf. Yesudian-Haich, *Yoga and Health*, Allen and Unwin.

dream, usually like a bad dream. He was not *there now*. He was not *awake*.

Now man begins to come alive, to grow conscious, to liberate himself from time and space. He feels the fire of life within him, he begins to become himself. Now he suddenly understands what Christ meant when he called some people 'dead' and some 'living'.

It is in fact as impossible to describe these states as it is to describe the taste of the chestnut. One can only speak in similes: expressions like: 'being awake', 'growing more conscious than hitherto', 'to come alive', and so forth, are substitutes for a non-existent, more adequate vocabulary. The best way of putting it is perhaps as follows: however convinced we may be that we were awake, conscious and *living*, we nevertheless only awake through the higher frequencies of creative power, and see then that we have been neither awake, conscious nor living, but that we have vegetated and led an unreal life. Just as, while we are dreaming, we are convinced that we are 'awake' and 'living' in our dream-visions, and we only realize that we have been dreaming when we 'wake up' to our normal consciousness, in the same way we only realize that we have hitherto led a dream-life – a shadow-life – when we gradually waken through the effect of the 'dragon-fire'. How superbly Andersen describes this state in his fairy-tale 'The Shadow' and Gustav Meyrink in his great book *Das Grüne Gesicht*.

When we experience this 'awakening' we cannot understand how we ever believed that we were awake and living. A much greater vitality has wakened in man, but its activity is not in the body, no heat whatever is felt (as some expect), but in the consciousness, in the spirit, we feel a fire within us, a *light*! A great many people who long for this 'awakening' try to experience it inwardly and make the great mistake in meditation of wanting to experience some mystical state *physically*. This is an error! Every one of these states is exclusively a *state of consciousness*. That is to say, that I myself am *the light of consciousness*, and the body is only involved in this inasmuch as it too begins to grow much more intensely alive. It is charged with new vitality, it grows younger and healthier. It becomes a submissive and obedient servant of one's own Self. We live in an intensified and sublime state. This state is not one of hysteria and paroxysm. On the contrary, we are in an intensified, clear, lucid, spiritual state of consciousness, and are much calmer than before. In a paroxysmal state we let ourselves go, losing control over our nerves and ourselves. In the spiritually elevated state, our *calmness, control and objectivity* are incomparably greater than previously in the normal state. Precisely because we are '*here now*', we are '*with ourselves*' to a much greater extent than we would ever have thought possible. In the spiritually illumined, awake state we are *calmness, self-control* itself. We are our own master, our own Self. That is true *presence of mind*, which we can sustain continuously as normal consciousness beyond the period of meditation. In this state we have no conscience, because we have become the conscience itself.

Meditators occasionally expect 'visitations' or 'visions', or they doze off perhaps in the belief that in meditation the higher Self will penetrate their consciousness like a strange being and provide them with another Self, another consciousness. They labour under a great misconception and in so doing reveal that they have no idea of true meditation – of SELF-realization. The truly spiritual states are very easy: one is simply *here now*! And completely awake, as awake as the clear light of the sun! This bright light is experienced in a perfectly clear, transparent conscious state of being as: I AM! We do not even think these two words, we *are* that without thinking words!

This state can also be achieved in work. Work absorbs man's attention, helps him to be 'here' and 'now', to be 'awake'. To the young man who asked him what he should do to be blessed, Christ replied simply: 'Watch and pray.' With that he said everything. And also when we work we awake and become ever more awake, if we devote ourselves to it with full concentration, full consciousness – but without thinking that we are 'conscious'. What kind of work ought it to be? Any kind. For the important thing is not *what* we work at, but how we work. Any kind of work, and that may include all kinds of sport or acrobatics, activities which require mastery of the mind over matter, the body. Anyone who has pursued a sport with full concentration and has gradually improved his performance will know the fervent and joyous states of mind which accompany mastery of the body. When a circus acrobat performs superhuman feats during his act, he experiences high spiritual rapture and joy. It is a well-known fact that some acrobats who risk their lives and those of their assistants during their act live ascetically like monks.

The pleasure and thrill experienced in their performances is infinitely greater than in a brief sexual encounter. *They even risk their lives for this higher kind of happiness.* (Something that a man would hardly do for a sexual experience.) Those who are friendly with circus people know that there are many among them who could say like Beethoven: 'There is no higher happiness than to achieve a victory over the body, or over wild animals and to demonstrate this victory of the mind – of the EGO – to men.'

Those whose work leaves them free time, or who are engaged anyway in an intellectual activity, can use this work for themselves as a ladder of consciousness – as Jacob's ladder. We should choose for ourselves whatever we have a liking for, what really interests us from the bottom of our hearts. It does not matter whether we sketch, paint, model, weave carpets or work Gobelins, play a musical instrument, go in for handicrafts or gardening, write poetry or books. One thing, however, is necessary, and that is that we must *never content ourselves with average achievements,* but always aim at perfection. There is nothing like creative work to facilitate progress and to help transform sexual energy into creative power and to radiate it as spiritual energy. Let us, then, work at something, whatever it may be. If we do so, we no longer need to worry about how to 'divert' our thoughts. They are absorbed in work, without the petty, personal awareness of the self. One is so closely bound up with the present that the thoughts, *always linking past with future,* cannot penetrate this *continuous present.* One automatically disconnects oneself from time and space. We direct sexual energy automatically and instinctively into the higher centres, where it operates as creative-magical powers. If we practise any kind of art, we must not worry about gaining recognition and fame. The source of this ambition is the little 'I', the person, who, although vain, at the same time lacks self-confidence and looks for acknowledgement, recognition from outside. We must not work in order to become 'recognized'. *The work* is the most essential thing, for we develop with it. Work for work's sake, for the sake of development, hastens our progress. The most important thing of all is *to concentrate fully on our work* – whatever it may be – *to be completely absorbed by it, and to enter into it heart and soul* and not to be easily satisfied, even if it is no more than simple housework. The true artist works for work's sake, he is happy while he is creating;

for him the work itself is the highest reward because while at work he is in an exalted, illumined state. To someone who throws himself wholeheartedly into his work, it makes absolutely no difference whether he is very gifted or starts at a lower level, for everything is merely relative. *We must try to rise from the stage we are at.* That is the most important thing of all. *To rise.* The greatest artist alive also had to start once at the lowest level, both as man and as artist, though this may have been a great many incarnations ago. If we lose no time and try to do our work as perfectly as possible by making every effort and applying our utmost concentration, then we shall learn that talents can grow quite unbelievably. Let us not be satisfied with inferior or mediocre work. Let us try to carry it out with even greater perfection and thoroughness so that we can bring out the most subtle nuances. Let us try to know our material thoroughly and to bring it under our yoke – which in Sanskrit is Yoga. We shall find that there is no limit to our powers of concentration. If we have been concentrating completely on our work until now, we discover on the next day that we can concentrate even more intensely and in the course of work fresh possibilities come to our knowledge, which previously had eluded us. We discover *the nature of work* and new, even more beautiful mysteries which we were hitherto unable to see, because we have again reached the next step in our development and our concentration has increased accordingly. New and wider worlds open before us, of which until now we knew as little as many other people. And yet all the time we were living in the midst of these worlds, but our eyes were still closed, still blind. Now, during work, we penetrate the innermost worlds right to the essential core of things and at the same time, also to *the core of our own being.* Outside our work, too, new worlds open before us. We suddenly begin to understand with great clarity writings of great men and prophets, which until now we had not understood properly, which we had found obscure and enigmatical. We are filled with unspeakable joy, we find new brothers, new friends, who speak to us from past centuries and millennia across time and space, to us, because we *understand* them, because we have become *one* with them.

And so we continue our work, especially on ourselves. We taste of the purely spiritual joys and raptures which are not to be compared with brief, physical pleasures. The undescribable delight of doing creative work fills our whole being with unutterable ecstasy both during the work and when we rest. Creative power continues to be active in us. We can scarcely wait to get down to work again, for we feel that only during work *do we really live*. Something within us has opened. Through the ever-increasing creative powers the joy of freedom and boundlessness has started to blossom. We have a strange feeling as if it were not we who are working, but something within us that knows everything, that takes us and shows us the way in which we can achieve and manifest perfect harmony, indeed, even perfection in our work. This something and I are completely one. And we understand what the Zen-Buddhists mean by 'Zen', and also the significance of the mystical marriage – *unio mystica* of the Rosicrucians and the great mystics – because we have experienced it within us during work and experience it still. I and the creative principle – *logos* – are *one*!

I – and I – are *one*!

A fever grips us, we forget the whole world, we are no longer a person who has a name somewhere in the outer world, for we have become a drop in the infinite ocean. We participate in God's creation and create new worlds, however small our own world, but we feel, we know, that we have the ability within us to reach, in our little sphere, a creative perfection comparable to that of God in the universe. The door to the inner world opens even wider, time and again we glimpse new worlds, new splendours. I discover new truths, I receive new ideas. Where from? From within MYSELF, where there is an inexhaustible source – from God. What is the difference? Is there one at all? These are all mere words. The ideas which become conscious in me are light like the shining light of God, and by this light I see everything, all the truths of heaven and earth, wherever I direct the reflector of my consciousness. This light fills me with unspeakable happiness and unutterable joy. The body also shares in these pleasures: in my heart, my breast, my head, the crown of my head and in every fibre of my nerves, I feel new, animating life which gives me vitality, courage, self-confidence – LIFE itself – so that I can no longer be afraid of anything, of anything at all. Not even of death. Divine, imperturbable peace prevails in me, I AM MYSELF this peace and self-confidence. I neither need nor expect a reason in order to be 'happy', because I *am* myself happiness. What *else*, then, could make me happy? I *am* the source from which happiness radiates. Am I conscious – or unconscious? What kind of words are these? What do they mean? These states stand above such concepts. I AM! Is not that enough? Indeed it is. *I am* in reality! I live! I *am* LIFE! Why should my consciousness also need to perceive that rationally and to register it? If I have become the chestnut itself, why write a dissertation on its taste – my taste – if I myself AM it? Do I need to think or talk about that, when I am alive as I have never been alive before? Is it not enough that I myself AM *joy, happiness,* BEING?

I do not need to ponder on that any longer, or even to think about it. Words such as the 'unconscious' or the 'conscious' are just words, but they are not what they *are*. The words are outside, in the outer world, external to my Self, somewhere in my brain. In my inner world there IS only MYSELF. And I do not think this either, and if I am doing so now it is only in order to write it down, to make it comprehensible, to put it into words for the people who are troubled by this question. *I am* in the inspiration of BEING, *I myself*, without thinking it, without puzzling over it. There is nothing else that could entice me out of my BEING. Time . . . space . . . these are concepts of the outer world. For me there exists only the absolute existence – BEING itself . . . because I AM IT.

We are as unable to describe and make others comprehend the state of *being*, as we are to explain how to hear a sound, to smell a perfume, taste a flavour, to see a colour or a shape. Those who have already experienced these things smile sympathetically because they know what one is talking about. The others can only do one thing: *experience it themselves*. Thus it is with the transformation of sexual energy into spiritual-divine powers. Anyone who has experienced it can smile sympathetically, and this smile is the well-known smile of the Buddha, who knows everything, who knows the highest truth, who knows the highest truth about God – about eternal BEING. . . . If we have not experienced it we cannot understand what it is in the transformation of sexual energy that yields such deep contentment as to make the effort worth while. How can one, for instance, explain to a creature born without sexual organs what makes a sexual experience so pleasurable that men are capable of the highest heroism as well as of the greatest madness for the sake of sexual intercourse with one particular person? One can only advise people who have not personally experienced the transformation of sexual energy, and who sneer with scorn and contempt, not to pass judgement or to make it the subject of bad jokes. They should first try to experience the transformation. They should consider why all the great men who have ever wanted to explain to us the divine truths about the way of man's liberation from the bondage of matter to the omnipotence of the spirit, have without exception preceded us on *this* path. These titanic minds have taught us that the attainment of consciousness in the highest centres where we *do not reflect* on something, but *become, are* something, is the highest, divine state. And the driving force helping us to this state is sexual energy which has not been used up in sexual experience but directed inwards and transformed into creative-divine energy. The serpent which bites its own tail! 'He that hath ears to hear, let him hear' (Mark 4:9).

And the body? Will sexual desires never again be roused in the body? How do the glands react?

One thing we must not forget: the body only has sexual desires if *I am within*. The body itself does not have sexual desires. These are the physical projection of my urge for divine unity. A corpse does not have sexual desires. If I have attained divine unity – the *unio mystica* – in my consciousness, that is to say, if I have become one with my spirit, my being, thus forming a whole, then I no longer project sexual desires in the body. The innermost, true being – the spirit – is sexless. My body calms down like a tamed animal obeying my every command, and yet, it *lives with much greater intensity* and has *much greater potency* than the body of a man who is still in the grip of sexuality and expends life-giving energy. With each sexual union living creatures die a little. Again and again they spend their own vital energy, whether or not the aim of giving life to a new creature is achieved. *If we have become a whole, all our vital energy remains in the service of our own body,* since we use and radiate spiritualized sexual energy, creative power, also through the body. Each small fibre of our nerves is charged with this highest of divine-magical currents. Thus we can understand why the majority of the great men who have preceded us on the long path to the goal, had very healthy bodies and lived to an exceptionally great age. We shall mention only two well-known examples: at the age of ninety, St Anthony begins to till the soil in the Sahara and harvests so much corn that henceforth he can live on it. At the age of 104 he visits St Paul, who is now 112. Anthony had to go on foot for more than two days in order to reach Paul. These are historical facts which the then Bishop of Alexandria had recorded. We could list many authentic examples of how great men who practised total asceticism remained healthy and capable of work right to the extreme limits of the human life-span. The important thing, however, is not to live long, but to live *healthily*. We need to look after our body only to the extent of keeping it healthy, in absolute equilibrium, in heavenly peace. Just as the sun pours its rays evenly into the room, so we, helped by the directing of consciousness, must radiate the energy, which is my EGO, which I AM, through all the nerve centres. For let us not forget that our sexual glands are intended not only for preservation of the species but that they also have the above-mentioned important part to play for our own body. They bear the vital tension in our body and the youthfulness of the latter is dependent upon this tension. Equilibrium, harmony, confidence and peace in my body – and I am master in my house. And man's greatest enemy, fear, cannot lay hold of me any more than darkness can lay hold of light.

Just as the spirit is a thousand times stronger than the flesh, the body, so too the happiness and joy attained by this way of life is a thousand times greater. The spirit is the cause, the body the effect. The body is a mere reflection of the spirit, and sexual enjoyment, even the highest sensual pleasure, is only a pale reflection of the joy, fulfilment, and bliss experienced through sexual energy converted into creative power – *logos* – and retained as a state of consciousness – since I AM IT. This happiness we do not expend only in order to let it build up and then to expend it again and again till the body is worn out, exhausted and impotent. We retain inner divine joy, we bear it within us all the time, we *ourselves are this joy*. And what is more, it keeps growing from day to day, just as in the fairy-tale the golden apple of love grows larger and larger the more one eats of it! Creative power, increased by concentration of the mind, keeps growing until we consciously reach the boundlessness of the divine Self. And the body participates in this heightening of the creative powers. It grows ever healthier from the higher frequencies of the expanding consciousness, it becomes ever more the submissive servant of the spirit. It rests with the individual how he uses his creative powers, expends them, administers them. Now we understand why those who reached the highest level, the prophets, the sibyls, the God-men, refrained from expending their creative powers as sexual energy. They were not foolish people who discarded a source of pleasure and enjoyment. They experienced the other pole consciously within them and therefore did not need to look for a complement outside. They complemented themselves, what had been a half became a WHOLE. Consciously, by themselves, they became the creative power – *logos* – their own divine *Self*.

That is the transformation of sexual energy into spiritual, divine-creative power. That is the resurrection from death to eternal LIFE. And the secret of sexual energy is this: to begin with, as the link between the world of matter and the spiritual realm, it helps the human spirit to be born into a material body – afterwards, however, it compels and helps man in his own efforts, using sexual energy as fuel, to stimulate his higher nerve and brain centres, thereby raising his consciousness to divine universal awareness, while still in the body. That is why we must take the opportunity during our earthly life, while we still live in the body, of attaining the ultimate goal of every living creature – God.

Let us use a simile: a piece of firewood yearns for the fire. It is cold, stiff and lifeless and longs to be warmed through. It longs to live, to be exalted. It longs for the divine fire. Then one day it is set alight, it starts burning and thus the wood becomes one with the fire which heats it, animates it and exalts it. But precisely because the fire heats it, and makes it alive, the wood burns up, turns to ash and dies. The wood does not realize that there is release from this death and the possibility of resurrection. If it made use of the time when it was alight to transmit its consciousness from itself to the fire, in order to become conscious in the latter, *to become* one, identical with the fire *itself*, when the wood died, its consciousness would *not* have to die also. In that case it would not matter to it whether the fire which it has now become burns further pieces of wood or not. As fire, it would have the chance to go on existing in its invisible, non-manifest, spiritual form even if the fire burnt nothing. With the fire, the consciousness of the former wood could then continue to exist in its new-born, resurrected true being, as FIRE.

Our path is the same. If we human beings realize that we do not inevitably die with the material body provided that we use the time and opportunity during our life, while we burn with the fire of the spirit, to transmit our consciousness from our human substance to the spirit, the burning fire – to life – then, when the body perishes, the consciousness will not die. As Paul says: 'We shall not all sleep, but we shall all be changed' (I Cor. 15:51).

We must, then, make use of the time and the opportunity so long as we live in the body, so long as the spirit quickens us and burns within us and our body is still in possession of its full potency. The spirit gives us life. Hence, if we consciously become identical with our fire, our spirit, while we still burn – while we still live – then we shall awake in life itself, grow conscious at a new level, that is to say, we shall become life itself, which can never die for the very reason that it is LIFE. At this point we ourselves have become the fire – the spirit – life – *logos* – which creates all things, animating and preserving them by its fire. In fact this is what we have always been except that our consciousness has fallen out of the spiritual, paradisiacal state into the 'wood', into the body, becoming identical with it. If, however, a person is not conscious in his true being, then his consciousness dies with his body and he is truly dead. If, on the other hand, he becomes conscious in his higher *Self*, in his spirit, during his earthly life, during his incarnation – as long as he burns with the fire of the spirit – then *his consciousness does not die with the body*. Instead, it remains conscious and lingers on like a drop of water in the ocean, in a state of universal consciousness, in God. The Christian definition of this is resurrection, the Oriental definition is nirvana. All the great prophets, sibyls and God-men who have lived in this world, have taught men that the attainment of this state of consciousness – the identification of the consciousness with life, with eternal BEING, with God – is the supreme goal, but one within our reach. This is the release from the laws of matter, of the body, the redemption from death and from the crucifixion of our spirit on the two great beams of time and space. This is the dawning of consciousness, the awakening in life itself, in God himself, redeemed from the unconscious spirit in the body. This resurrection in the new consciousness is the teaching of Christ, of the Eastern philosophies of Yoga and religion, of the medieval alchemists, the Rosicrucians, of all past and present religions and of every great initiate. This is the core of every religion, for there is only *one* truth and *one* secret of our being. All initiates have seen and taught the very same truth, even if in accordance with race and climatic conditions of their particular country they have concealed the essence of their doctrines in the most varied disguises. Through the variety of religions we have also been taught various paths – conditioned by the disposition and nature of the individual peoples. The shortest path to God, however, namely stimulating the higher nerve and brain centres with sexual energy as 'fuel', and thereby laying hold of the magical powers which can only be developed from a youthful, virile body, was taught in Europe in the sixteenth and seventeenth centuries by the so-called alchemists, the Rosicrucians. The Crusades were the real occasion for their acquiring the knowledge of the Oriental initiates about the philosopher's stone. They spoke of an athanor, in which the fire had to burn continuously and steadily in order to produce the philosopher's stone. From their writings and ingenious illustrations, it is perfectly evident that they produced this stone out of man himself. The athanor is the human body, the dragon is the creative power which works in the body, and the dragon's fire is sexual energy directed upwards through an abstemious way of life and used as fuel. The philosopher's stone is the divine universal consciousness and its magical-spiritual power over the whole of Nature. And the elixir of life is the 'fire which flows like water', 'the fiery water', that is to say, the high frequencies of divine self-awareness which we can conduct into the body and radiate as consciously as we can conduct electricity and magnetism into a piece of metal, thus charging it and making it magnetic. Christians call this current 'the blood of Christ', the Rosicrucians call it the 'elixir of life'. This is the vital current of the *logos*, of life, of the divine Self.

The great initiates, prophets, sibyls, high priests and priestesses of the great peoples of the past, and the God-men who from time to time have appeared on earth, were and are not foolish people. They would not have thrown away the sexual pleasures which very many people regard as the be-all and end-all of life, if they had not received in exchange something a thousand times more valuable. They merely exchanged the 'wood' for the fire. As initiates, they calmly sacrificed these physical, very brief, transient pleasures for the source of all joy and happiness, for the eternal and everlasting being of all potency, which is the giver of bliss, freedom and omnipotence. What is our preference? The geyser that shoots up now and again, or the volcano bubbling in the bowels of the earth, which is the source and cause of all geysers and volcanic eruptions?!

The mystical marriage, also described in the Bible in the Song of Solomon and in the Apocalypse, is the union of the human consciousness with the true Self, with the divine spirit, through the help of spiritualized sexual energy.

In the classic fairy-tale of *Sleeping Beauty*, we find the same truth. The Sleeping Beauty (the sleeping consciousness) is wakened to eternal life through the power of love (through the fire of sexual energy) by the prince's *kiss* (by the fiery touch of the spirit, of true being).

The Siegfried legend has the same meaning. Siegfried conquers the dragon with the sword of consciousness, then bathes in the dragon's blood, which gives him eternal life and magical-supernatural powers. Then he steps through the ring of fire surrounding the sleeping Brunhilde, and with a kiss – like the prince in *Sleeping Beauty* – wakens her to eternal life and everlasting union. The two poles find each other, to rest again within each other in absolute equilibrium.

We could quote many more symbolical tales and legends which relate the same secret of the awakening of the human consciousness to eternal, divine universal awareness through the fire of retained sexual energy. But that would take us too far. The fact is that man has this potential within him, even if he is totally unaware of it. God dwells in man's unconscious, and, as already mentioned, the two poles rest within each other in God. Man thinks and lives sexually only as long as he identifies his consciousness with his body. If, however, he awakens in God with his consciousness, then the sexual mentality and concept of the sexes ceases to exist in him. In himself, in the revealed, and as a result, now conscious unconscious (which in this state is precisely no longer an unconscious), he finds the other pole – his own complement, which had always been there, but in a latent, unconscious condition – and he becomes one with it. Now, since *everything* has become conscious in him – in the first person – in me, so that I no longer have an unconscious, the other pole has become conscious in me, and I realize that *I myself am* it as well. In the partner of the opposite sex with whom I felt an inner unity and tried to experience and realize this also in the body, I sought this complement – which like the Sleeping Beauty was latent and dormant within me – of my absolute, true Self, in which both poles have always rested and will continue to do so to all eternity, because they belong together, because I MYSELF AM both parts. When we have attained the divine unity of complete universal consciousness, we are conscious in the absolute *androgynous* state. The Rosicrucians called a person who had achieved this state, a hermaphrodite. The word is composed of the two Greek names Hermes and Aphrodite, and means that the person has realized the two poles in his *consciousness*. In the depiction of this, the Rosicrucians showed the 'hermaphrodite' with two heads, because he has achieved his illumined state through mastery of sexual energy, used as fuel, and they placed him on a dragon, the ruler of this world, of our earth. For sexual energy rules on earth.

All of man's various holy writings speak of this androgynous or hermaphroditic primal state. In the Bible it is represented in the story of Adam, who, to begin with, was an androgynous creature, a man-woman. Not until Adam fell into a deep sleep – that is to say when he had lost his divine state of consciousness and become an unconscious creature – did the negative pole, the female principle, leave his body. Then God made 'coats of skins and clothed them' (Gen. 3:21), that is to say, their spirit clothed itself in a material body, which manifests only *one* sex, and thus they also acquired *sexual awareness*. They imagined themselves to be man and woman and forgot that their Self is SPIRIT and a WHOLE.

The present order of Nature does not allow us to attain or realize physically the androgynous primal state. This is only possible in the spiritual state, in the primal consciousness. We can achieve and experience this divine primal state in which the two poles rest within each other, *in our consciousness* as a *state of consciousness*.

It is necessary to stress that a man's body continues in the same way to belong to a sex when he has already reached the very highest level. If, through Yoga exercises, we render conscious the other, latent half of our being and realize our complement within us, our body still remains male *or* female and on no account a man-woman, a physical hermaphrodite. Under the present order of Nature that would be an abnormal, pathological condition of the body. The Rosicrucians, then, used the expression 'hermaphrodite' only with reference to the consciousness. All the states which we experience in the course of our development are *purely states of consciousness*. And when we have made the other sex also conscious in ourselves, this nevertheless remains a purely *mental state*. The body is only involved inasmuch as it no longer has sexual desires. Desire is not in the body – as we have said already, a corpse does not have sexual desires – but in man's state of consciousness, as long as he identifies himself with the body. At the time of conception, the spirit falls into the body, builds the body for itself in its image and makes it alive. Since matter isolates and does not admit the light of the spirit, the latter loses its spiritual consciousness, becomes a physical being and imagines itself to be a body. As a result, it projects its search for the lost unity into the body, thereby giving rise to sexual desire in the body. For the glands are stimulated and work also through the effect of the spirit, of life. When the spirit regains its spiritual consciousness in the body and becomes aware of being spirit, it then becomes a *whole* in its consciousness, and sexual desire ceases in the body as well. That is the secret which explains why men who are awake in the spirit, in their true being – the saints, prophets, sibyls and God-men – no longer have sexual desires, although their bodies also manifest only one sex, and it explains why they are able to lead an abstemious life without pathological repression, restlessness and difficulties. To avoid any misunderstanding, let me emphasize that through becoming a *'whole'*, these enlightened men did not become impotent, no matter how often ignorant people may claim the contrary. Those who have reached the goal have become the source of all potency, they use their energies as they please, and the door to every manifestation – and that includes sexual manifestations – is open before them. They are, then, not impotent, but balanced, harmonious, perfectly calm and controlled men. Each one of us carries these truths and laws in his unconscious.

We seek the absolute. We cannot accept compromises. And why not? *Because we already bear this 'absolute', this 'whole', within us, because we ourselves have been this since primeval times and still are.* Our 'EGO' is pure spirit, for which there exists no kind of division, separation and splitting into the two sexes. When we have grown conscious in our true Self, all sexuality falls from us like a ripe fruit from a tree, just as the child, when it is grown-up, gives up playing with tin-soldiers painlessly and without sacrifice. And the body obeys us, since sexual energy no longer irritates the glands. It is used as creative power through other, higher centres. Each man can experience these facts himself if he tries to progress on the path described here, which is the shortest one.

We must never be afraid that God would take something away from us without giving us something much greater in return. HE lives in us as our innermost being, as our true Self, it is HIS wish to realize himself in our mortal humanity. As long as we are unconscious living creatures, God lives in our immeasurably great, boundless *unconscious*. And if we have grown completely conscious within ourselves, God lives in us as our own divine EGO.

He that hath an ear, let him hear what the Spirit saith . . . TO HIM THAT OVERCOMETH WILL I GIVE TO EAT OF THE TREE OF LIFE, WHICH IS IN THE MIDST OF THE PARADISE OF GOD . . . BE THOU FAITHFUL UNTO DEATH, AND I WILL GIVE THEE A CROWN OF LIFE (Rev. 2:7, 10).

# Conclusion

Let us try to summarize what has been said in order to put it into perspective.

There is only one creative energy – *logos* – which manifests itself from its lowest form, sexual energy, to the supreme spiritual-divine power, to all-consciousness, through the whole scale of creation at all levels of the great Jacob's ladder, in the macrocosm, in the universe, as in the microcosm, in man.

Man has the inborn ability to consciously manifest creative power in all its forms, at all levels of creation, since creative power – *logos* – is his own, true Self and he has in his body the organs capable of radiation which correspond to the various forms of energy.

Earthly life normally urges man to raise his consciousness ever higher, to ever more spiritual levels, to grow ever more aware till he finally attains divine all-consciousness. This is the purpose of his life, of his incarnation. Yet, this normal course takes a very long time, it is laborious and fraught with pain and sorrow. Man, however, carries within him, in his body, a secret. Once he has realized that, he will be able greatly to shorten the long path to consciousness and to quicken his development, so that he is capable of achieving this goal in one single life. The secret is, that in order to reach the highest goal, he can accelerate the stimulation and activation of his nerve and brain centres, already built into the body, but still in a latent condition, by a living fire. The living fire is his own sexual energy. This energy is the link between mind and matter, through it a living body emerges from matter, because it helps the spirit into matter. In the same way, however, sexual energy allows the spirit the opportunity while still in the body of rising from its physical, graduated consciousness and returning again to God, to divine all-consciousness. Sexual energy bears within itself the faculty of quickening the development of the human consciousness to resurrection, to immortality, to divine all-consciousness. Sexual energy itself is transformed into creative-spiritual power, and man experiences this transformation within himself as continuously increasing, purely spiritual states of consciousness. He becomes ever more awake, alive and conscious. He becomes completely alert. At the same time, higher, spiritual-magical abilities develop in him.

The secret of sexual energy, therefore, is not only that it is capable of begetting new generations, but that it has a second function of much greater importance for man: to lead his consciousness step by step up the great Jacob's ladder of consciousness to God. In so doing, sexual energy, which is the creative principle itself – *logos* – is transformed into its original primal state. This transformation of creative energy from its lowest form, sexual energy, into its very highest form, into spiritual-divine vitality, can be consciously accelerated by man with the help of sexual energy. This is because sexual energy alone can help him to increase the resilience of his higher nerve and brain centres, still resting in a latent condition, to such an extent that they can tolerate the highest frequencies of divine self-awareness without detrimental effects.

Man experiences within himself the lowest form of creative power – called sexual energy – as an unconscious, physical-sexual urge for release; at the very highest level, as a purely spiritual state, as divine-universal love and as divine *all-consciousness* – as I AM.

From the lowest level at which man is still an animal plus reason, to the highest, divine-spiritual level, to universal consciousness, man ascends the seven rungs of the Jacob's ladder of consciousness. These are:

First level: man is still an unconscious creature, blindly driven by fate. His sex life is an animal, indiscriminate urge for release.

Second level: first dawn of consciousness, first awakening. In his sex life, search for a partner physically suited to him, already involving selection.

Third level: consciousness in emotional life. Search for activity suited to him emotionally, and in his sex life, for a partner suited to him spiritually, emotionally but also physically. Urge and yearning for a family unit.

Fourth level: consciousness at the intellectual level, thirst for knowledge, urge to study, search for intellectual occupation and work. In sex life, search for an intelligent, understanding partner suited to him in every respect, whom he marries for love.

Fifth level: awakening of the magical, suggestive powers, accordingly, creative activity and superior, suggestive effect on other people. Self-control and mastery of destiny. Search for embodiment of the complement present in the unconscious, for the partner suited to him intellectually, spiritually and physically. On the one hand, complete freedom from all the bourgeois conventions and laws of society, on the other, a morally superior outlook and way of life, motivated *by an inner urge*, and obeying *inner, divine laws of conscience.*

Sixth level: universal love, prophetic, priestly vocation, purely spiritual manifestations as a *whole*. A spiritual unity – mystical marriage – with one's own higher SELF, with the whole living world.

Seventh level: universal consciousness, *unio mystica* – man's consciousness unites with his true being – the Lamb and the new Jerusalem have become one. Consciousness in being, in God: '*I and my father are one.*'

In *one* human life man cannot pass through all these stages – from the lowest to the highest. For his nerves could not tolerate the vast difference of tension between the lowest and highest states of consciousness, although they have an unsuspected resilience. Man requires a very long time to cover the lower levels in order to increase the resistance of the nerves by degrees; to do so, he must have many reincarnations. But from the middle level, at which he is already awakened and wishes to progress consciously, to the highest level, he is capable of developing in a single human lifetime. With the help of the sexual energy present in his body, he can reach this level at a quickened pace, in a much shorter time than if he develops naturally. As soon as he ceases to expend sexual energy, retaining it instead as living fuel for himself, in order to stimulate and activate his nerve and brain centres still resting in a latent condition, he attains mastery over the spiritual-magical powers and obtains the goal of his life, all-consciousness in God.

He is helped to this goal on the shortened path by the deliberate performance of appropriate Yoga exercises handed down to us over thousands of years, and by sexual energy, which has not been expended, but used as inner fuel.

The sorrows of death compassed me, and the pains of hell gat hold upon me: I found trouble and sorrow.

I called upon the Lord in distress: the Lord answered me. . . . The Lord is on my side; I will not fear. . . . The Lord is my strength and song, and is become my salvation.

Return unto thy rest, O my soul; for the Lord hath dealt bountifully with thee.

For thou hast delivered my soul from death, mine eyes from tears, and my feet from falling.

Our soul is escaped as a bird out of the snare of the fowlers: the snare is broken, and we are escaped.

I will walk before the Lord in the land of the living (Psalms 116–124).

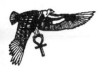 # INITIATION
## ELISABETH HAICH
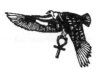

Written at the request of her advanced students, *Initiation* is an illuminating autobiography that connects the twentieth century European life of internationally beloved teacher Elisabeth Haich and her lucid memories of initiation into the hidden mystical teachings of the priesthood in ancient Egypt. A compelling story within a story emerges detailing the life experiences that catalyzed her spiritual path.

In an earlier life in ancient Egypt, a young woman is prepared for initiation into the esoteric secrets of the priesthood by the High Priest Ptahhotep, who instructs her step-by-step, consistent with her development, in the universal truths of life. Throughout this extraordinary book, Elisabeth Haich reveals her in depth insights into the subtle workings of karma, reincarnation, the interconnectedness of individual daily life choices and spiritual development Elisabeth Haich shares usually hidden truths that only a few rare individuals in any generation, seek, find and communicate to others, enabling the reader to awaken within the essential understanding necessary to enlighten any life no matter what events manifest.

In twentieth century Europe, from childhood to adulthood, through war and remarkable meetings, she demonstrates the power of turning the searchlight of one's consciousness inward and using every life event towards expanding consciousness.

*Initiation* is a timeless classic communicated in modern terms inspiring generations of spiritual seekers globally. Whether read as an autobiographical novel unveiling mystical truths or as a unique glimpse into Elizabeth Haich's exceptional journey to initiation, the personal impact on the reader is profound.

To read *Initiation* is to be part of the initiation itself.

ISBN:0-943358-50-7   Paperback   5½x 8½   376 Pages          $19.95

# THE DAY WITH YOGA

## Inspirational Words To Guide Daily Life

### Elizabeth Haich

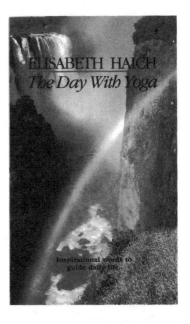

T hrough her best selling books —*Initiation, Sexual Energy and Yoga,* and *Wisdom of the Tarot*—Elisabeth Haich is internationally famous for her ability to assist others on their paths of spiritual unfoldment.

A unique creative energy is available each day of the week. Nature, all living creatures, plants, and human beings are deeply influenced by these subtle variations. We all bathe, float and are affected by the power operating that day.

Each Day is related to a specific planetary energy:

| | |
|---|---|
| Sunday—The Sun | Wednesday—Mercury |
| Monday—The Moon | Thursday—Jupiter |
| Tuesday—Mars | Friday—Venus |
| Saturday—Saturn | |

*The Day With Yoga,* is Elisabeth Haich's personal collection of meditation quotes. Each has been carefully selected to inspire and attune us to the vibration of the day, and to release a deeper level of harmony and inner peace into our lives.

ISBN: 0-943358-12-4      Paper      4×7      104 Pages

# SELF HEALING, YOGA & DESTINY

## Elisabeth Haich & Selvarajan Yesudian

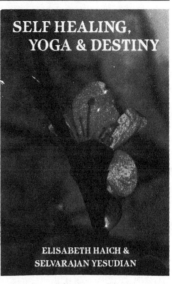

SELF HEALING, YOGA & DESTINY

ELISABETH HAICH & SELVARAJAN YESUDIAN

Through her best selling books, such as *Initiation*, Elisabeth Haich has become world famous for her profound understanding of the human soul. The Yoga schools she set up with Selvarajan Yesudian, have become internationally renowned. Designed to reconnect you with the Divine, the concepts in this book explain the attitudes necessary for the path back to one's self. Based on many years personal experience, the authors create an understanding of how to realize the essential source of life.

Learn Elisabeth Haich & Yesudian's personal views on:

- Love
- Suffering
- Destiny
- Illness
- Accidents
- Karma
- Black & White Magic
- Self Healing & Transformation

A wealth of insightful information is contained in this book to help you gain an expanded view of your life and consciousness.

> *"When we look about us in our daily living, we see how greatly people suffer in the chains they have forged for themselves, even when they are filled with longing for freedom. Is there any way for man to be free? To be free is to be free from the deceptive magic of the material world."*
>
> **HAICH AND YESUDIAN**

ISBN: 0-943358-06-X     Paperback     5½×8½     90 Pages

# WISDOM OF THE TAROT

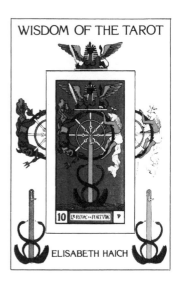

**WISDOM OF THE TAROT**

ELISABETH HAICH

**W**isdom of the Tarot relates the path to higher consciousness through the color, shape and symbolic forms on the twenty-two Tarot cards. Detailed study and meditation of each card may release internally all that is involved with each level encountered on the journey towards the Light. These cards may be used in conjunction with the text or separately for meditation. When studied individually, a card can reveal the necessary steps that need to be taken to actualize one's potential.

Tarot cards, or symbolic representations of the truth have always been used to help man relate not only with the mind, but internally, through the feelings invoked by the colors and forms. The nature of these cards is that they can produce a strong awakening of one's unconscious forces. They are like a spiritual mirror in which we can recognize and examine ourselves. We can then understand that the reasons for our fate lie within ourselves, and changes by the mere fact that we begin to react differently to everything that happens to us. These cards with the text are a valuable key to understand our present state, our past and in a deeper sense, how we create our future. Included within the book are pages of five color Tarot cards.

*"Elisabeth Haich has produced a masterly work of initiation into the secrets of life. Out of a deep understanding of being and her own intimate experience of union with her genius, she has illustrated the process by which man becomes man by his insight into the pictures of the twenty two rungs of the ladder of divine ascent, on which each rung is an experience for the next rung in accordance with the individual's plan of life."*

**DR. EWALT KLIEMKE**

**ISBN: 0-943358-01-9**     **Paperback**     **6×9**     **174 Pages**

# The Planetarization of Consciousness

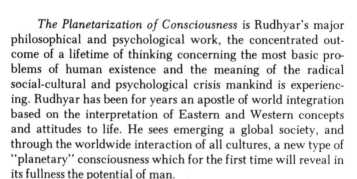

### by Dane Rudhyar

*The Planetarization of Consciousness* is Rudhyar's major philosophical and psychological work, the concentrated outcome of a lifetime of thinking concerning the most basic problems of human existence and the meaning of the radical social-cultural and psychological crisis mankind is experiencing. Rudhyar has been for years an apostle of world integration based on the interpretation of Eastern and Western concepts and attitudes to life. He sees emerging a global society, and through the worldwide interaction of all cultures, a new type of "planetary" consciousness which for the first time will reveal in its fullness the potential of man.

*"The holistic world-view which I present here is meant to be an incentive to think greater thoughts, to feel deeper, more inclusive feelings, and to act as "agents" for the Power that structures human evolution—however we wish to image this power."*

*The Planetarization of Consciousness* is essentially an act of faith in Man. Man as a microcosm of the universe, Man as a reality that transcends the physical organism, all localisms and nationalisms, and in whom spirit and matter can unite in a "Divine Marriage" productive of ever new and greater creative tomorrows.

Rudhyar, an accomplished and innovative painter, composer, poet, astrologer and philosopher has actualized a "humanistic" yet deeply spiritual approach to existence.

Paper 320 pp.

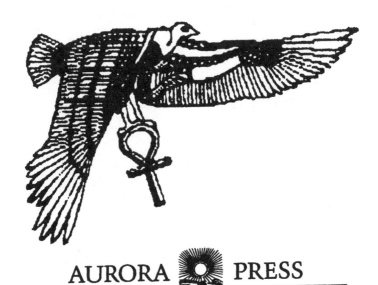

## AURORA PRESS

For our online catalog
& ordering info, visit,
www.AuroraPress.com

Aurora Press
PO Box 573
Santa Fe, N.M. 87504

Fax 505 982-8321
www.AuroraPress.com
Email: Aurorep@aol.com

Credit Card Orders Only
Fax  734 995-8535
Tel.  888 894-8621